Designer Children

Designer Children

Reconciling Genetic Technology, Feminism, and Christian Faith

Karen Peterson-Iyer

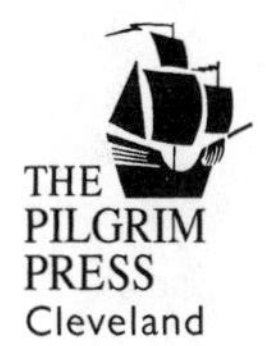

Cleveland

For Alex and Chris

The Pilgrim Press, 700 Prospect Avenue
Cleveland, Ohio 44115-1100, U.S.A.
thepilgrimpress.com

Printed in the United States of America on acid-free paper

09 08 07 06 05 04 5 4 3 2 1

Library of Congress Cataloging-in-Publication Data

Petersen-Iyer, Karen.
Designer children : reconciling genetic technology, feminism, and Christian faith / Karen Petersen-Iyer.
p. cm.
Includes bibliographical references and index.
ISBN 0-8298-1611-9 (pbk. : alk. paper)
1. Human reproductive technology – Moral and ethical aspects. 2. Human reproductive technology – Religious aspects – Christianity. 3. Genetic engineering – Moral and ethical aspects. 4. Genetic engineering – Religious aspects – Christianity. 5. Feminism. I. Title.
RG133.5.P488 2004
176 – dc22

2004054777

Contents

Preface

In some ways, parents have always faced the question of how much to intervene in their children's lives: how much to shape the directions they take and how much to let children choose their own paths. Yet the progression of technology has put a new spin on this age-old question and has lifted up new — and potentially much more powerful — ways that parents might begin to "shape" their children, even at the fundamental level of the human gene.

The development of technologies that may eventually enable us to "design" children offers both unprecedented chances for furthering human well-being and unprecedented dangers for placing that well-being in jeopardy. We as a society will need to make choices about how to approach and utilize these technologies — choices that we will make in our bedrooms, in our boardrooms, in our clinics, and in the halls of our legislatures. My hope is to begin to construct some moral ground under our feet as we do so. To this end, I draw upon the best insights from Christian faith and from feminist thought to begin to evaluate various ways of genetically "shaping" children. My own experiences as a parent obviously color my perspectives and are woven into my analyses. It is my belief that, although the force of technology may appeal to our instinct to protect procreative liberty at all costs, we must instead consider certain limits on the genetic "shaping" of children if we are to preserve and foster human well-being. These pages begin to explore what those limits should be.

As with any work of length, numerous persons have supported this project from behind the scenes, without whom it never would have been successfully completed. First, I wish to thank several friends and colleagues who extended critical support at various junctures: Christopher

Steck, S.J., Diana C. Gibson, and David Clough offered sustained encouragement, gently challenged my ideas, and provided technical help where needed. My own parents, Nancy and Donald Peterson, provided me with the steadfast support I needed on so many occasions; I also credit them with planting the first seeds of my feminist spirit, which I count as central to who I am.

I wish to thank my editor at Pilgrim Press, Pamela Johnson, who from the beginning has been an enthusiastic and inspiring voice. In addition, the librarians at the National Reference Center for Bioethics Literature at Georgetown University were immensely helpful at various points throughout my research.

I also offer thanks to several mentors and colleagues who, throughout the many steps leading up to this book, offered guidance, words of wisdom, and encouragement. In particular, Gene Outka, Karen Lebacqz, LeRoy Walters, and Catherine Bell proved to be worthy mentors and have helped me in various ways to begin and/or continue the lengthy process of scholarship. I am especially grateful to Gene as well as to Serene Jones and Thomas Ogletree for reading the first draft of the manuscript and offering helpful suggestions.

Finally, I owe a special debt of gratitude to two people. First is mentor and friend Margaret Farley, whose faith, patience, wisdom, and brilliance continue to amaze and inspire me; a finer ethicist there has not been. Second is Mohan S. Iyer, whose tremendous support at every step fortifies me in ways too numerous to name. Both of these people have helped me more fully to experience the many dimensions of Nelle Morton's wonderful phrase "hearing each other to speech."

This book is gratefully and lovingly dedicated to my own children, Alex and Chris, who have taught me deeply about myself, about faithful parenting, and about the miracle that God offers us in the gift of a child.

Introduction

Freedom, Control, and the Shaping of Children

IN ONE SENSE, the history of humanity is the history of having children. The processes of human procreation — the begetting, bearing, and rearing of children — together make up a central thread of the human story. Until the relatively recent past, these processes were in large part, though certainly not entirely, beyond human control. However, the advent of relatively safe and widely available birth control and medically assisted abortion has significantly increased the measure of human control over whether and when to procreate: procreation has become a genuine choice. Science has not stopped there, however; powerful new reproductive and genetic technologies have begun to change the face of human reproduction at an even more fundamental level, opening up reproduction to the coitally infertile and even making possible direct human influence over the genetic makeup of children themselves. For the first time in human history, couples soon may be able directly to preselect or alter certain genetic characteristics of their offspring.

This final technological development is my central concern in the pages that follow, for it opens up new horizons in procreation whereby parents will begin to exercise an unprecedented level of control over the type of children they have. To be sure, many scientists today issue repeated reassurances that we are nowhere near the level of genetic control that science fiction has presaged. Nevertheless, the prospect of "designer children"[1] — children free from serious genetic "defect" or with other deliberately selected physical or mental characteristics —

looms in the future, inspiring both awe and fear on the part of ethicists and lay persons alike. Indeed, the tremendous power of such genetic technologies, and their potential to be used either for good or for evil, is of urgent moral concern. Their availability no doubt will affect the way we think about children, about the women who bear them, and about the human body and the meaning of human reproduction itself.

In the United States contemporary ethical discussion has centered on the norm of procreative liberty as a way to make sense of, and make normative decisions about, these genetic technologies. This has been particularly true of liberal theorists, who in general have granted a highly privileged status to an individual's (or a couple's) prerogative in making reproductive choices. Moreover, the importance of procreative liberty in human fulfillment has been raised to a level of critical awareness by many contemporary feminists who see its guarantee as a modern milestone on the road to a world less oppressive for women. Hence, both liberal theorists and contemporary feminists contribute to the insight that procreative liberty can and should play a key role in determining what genetic technologies will mean and how they will be used.

Yet the argument I make here, critiquing a strongly liberal stance, is that procreative liberty is problematic when it is too heavily weighted in the evaluation of the genetic manipulation of offspring characteristics. Although it is an extremely important norm, procreative liberty itself must be moderated and situated more squarely into the broader context of human flourishing, taking account of key elements of our relational and common life. *My claim is that the norm of human flourishing, rather than simply that of procreative liberty, must guide us as we wade through the morass of ethical questions surrounding genetic manipulation.* Here I draw insight from both feminist and Christian sources in order to compose such a portrait of human flourishing.

When applied to the particular issue of "designer children," the constraints associated with this vision of human flourishing should lead us to affirm certain forms of genetic manipulation, to reject others outright, and, with still others, to exercise extreme caution. Along these lines, throughout this work I examine three particular instances of possible efforts to control the genetic qualities of offspring: the genetic prevention of cystic fibrosis, the genetic enhancement of memory, and preconceptive sex selection. My *contention is that, provided certain conditions are met, the practice of genetic manipulation to prevent serious disease generally should be embraced; that in all but rare situations the genetic enhancement of memory should be rejected; and that we should approach preconceptive sex selection with extreme caution and, in most cases, a bias toward discouragement.*

To arrive at these conclusions, I begin by locating the topic of genetic manipulation within a scientific and moral landscape, examining the procedures involved and probing the perceived benefits and dangers of genetic manipulation. Any informed discussion of genetic manipulation must include some basic scientific understanding of how such manipulation may be achieved, and this is part of the aim of the first chapter. Moreover, since the terms "genetic manipulation," "genetic engineering," or even "designer children" are not always used in a uniform way in today's public discussion, here I pinpoint how the three forms of manipulation I have chosen fit into the overall scientific picture. The chapter concludes with a general introduction to some of the more commonly raised ethical concerns encircling the issue.

In the second chapter I discuss some key aspects of sociocultural context that constitute an important backdrop to such genetic manipulation. First among these is the contemporary tendency to maintain increasingly perfectionist attitudes toward children. In the latter part of the chapter I move to an even more troubling aspect of the context of genetic manipulation: the historical promotion of eugenic thought and practices within Western society. Given the common "slippery slope" fears that surround the use of genetic technologies today, this history and social context cannot responsibly be ignored.

In the third and fourth chapters I canvass various sources for insight about the genetic manipulation of offspring. Chapter 3 first examines strong proponents of procreative liberty coming from what is traditionally considered a "liberal" perspective, which arguably dominates U.S.

public debate today. The second part of the chapter considers a feminist critique of these views, which, I argue, too strongly privilege procreative liberty at the expense of human well-being. In the fourth chapter I consider the insights that Christian theology and ethics offer on the subject of genetic manipulation. In spite of a wide variety of approaches to the topic, all bearing the name "Christian," the tradition carries within it several key themes and arguments that shed light on the issues related to genetic manipulation.

Together, the views examined in chapters 3 and 4 begin to point toward a vision of human flourishing, one broader than a narrow-minded focus on procreative liberty allows. In chapter 5, then, I draw upon what I consider to be the key insights of these various views, along with insights offered in more specific accounts of human well-being, to arrive at my own normative portrait of human flourishing with respect to the genetic manipulation of children. Thus, rather than embracing procreative liberty as an unmitigated good, I believe that we must recognize its value as a part of human well-being and co-creativity, even while placing it within a broader account of human reproduction with an emphasis on human flourishing. In the final chapter I return more explicitly to the three specific forms of genetic manipulation that serve as examples throughout the entire work: genetic manipulation for the prevention of cystic fibrosis, for memory enhancement, and for sex preselection; I examine each of these in light of this more comprehensive vision of human flourishing.

My aim throughout this investigation is to provide an analysis that helps to further our common wisdom about this complex and difficult issue. Since my sources include explicitly feminist and Christian writers, I expect that such an undertaking will be of particular interest to feminists and to Christians, and that my conclusions will carry stronger normative weight for those audiences. However, I firmly believe that the insights that feminism and Christianity have to offer on this issue will also be illuminative for a broader discussion. In addition, my discussion is (except where explicitly noted) limited primarily to Western societies, and especially to the United States, where the concept of procreative liberty carries a substantial amount of weight in the public mindset. Though I hope that my conclusions will prove relevant to other societies as well, I do not pretend to understand them in the same depth that I do my own.

I should note at the outset that this inquiry is concerned primarily with *prospective* genetic manipulation. It does not undertake in any detailed way the issue of abortion for purposes of genetic selection. Ultimately the relevant technological developments, if perfected, likely will obviate the desire for such abortions; the "choosing" will occur at an earlier stage. Because the issue of abortion involves significantly different, albeit related, questions than those raised by other forms of genetic manipulation or selection, I believe that it is wise to bracket that issue in the present work.

I also note here that this work focuses primarily on the moral analysis of genetic manipulation of offspring characteristics; it does not undertake to provide detailed legal recommendations. Certainly the question of what the law should allow is a crucial one. However, what is morally desirable and what is legally permissible are conceptually separable issues, and I believe that before we can adequately address the latter, we must gain increased clarity on the former.

The prospect of genetically crafting our children is both fascinating and terrifying to most of us. It is crucial to remember that many of the scenarios that we might envision — for example, parents who "order up" the child of their choice — simply do not belong to the realm of the technologically possible. Nevertheless, it is imperative that careful ethical reflection about the prospect of "designer children" be done now, *before* such technologies are developed, so that the technologically possible does not become confused with the morally desirable. Indeed, even if we believe that full-fledged "designer children" are still a long way off, the ethical issues raised are sufficiently urgent and challenging to merit our attention; we as a society must begin to think about the ways in which we do, and do not, wish to walk down the paths that genetic technologies may open up to us. My hope here is to contribute to this reflective process and, in so doing, to urge on and broaden the discussion. Both feminism and Christianity have the potential to open our eyes to insights not often encountered in the popular or scientific press, insights about what it means to flourish — as parents, as human individuals, and as members of a rich and diverse human community. We will be a better society for considering such insights.

Notes

1. The term "designer children" is a contentious one. Some argue that it may sensationalize the prospects of genetic manipulation beyond what is or will be realistically feasible. I find it to be a provocative term, one that presses the central question of this work: to what degree should we as individuals and as a society allow ourselves to "shape" our children genetically? Though indeed the possibility of full control over — or, the ability to truly "design" — our children in all likelihood will never materialize, one might still understand certain efforts to genetically manipulate offspring characteristics as one form of "designing" children.

Chapter One

The Manipulation of Genes

In the United States today we tend to venerate scientific advance, to look to science for ultimate explanations for the mysteries of the universe. Nowhere is this more true than in the area of human genetics. The lofty words of James Watson, former head of the National Institute of Health's Center for Human Genome Research, express this tendency well: "We can have at our disposal the ultimate tool for understanding ourselves at the molecular level.... We used to think our fate is in our stars. Now we know, in large measure, our fate is in our genes."[1] Indeed, such high expectations are not atypical in the field of human genetics; the human genome has at times even been referred to as a modern-day "holy grail" of biology.

Whether or not such bold assertions are warranted (and there is substantial evidence, as we will see, that they are not), it cannot be denied that genes play a crucial role in the makeup of the human person — that is, in determining *why* we are *how* we are. To understand adequately the genetic manipulation of children, and ultimately the prospects for "designing" them, it first is necessary to grasp the essential structure of genes and their function in human heredity. Hence, the first part of this chapter is devoted to this scientific basis for genetic manipulation, as well as to a brief overview of contemporary efforts to understand and manipulate the human genome. I will also introduce three chosen examples of genetic manipulation, describing how each fits into the overall scientific picture of genetic manipulation. In the latter part of the chapter I will delve more deeply into the perceived benefits and dangers, from an ethical standpoint, of these three forms of genetic manipulation. I will return to these three specific forms of genetic manipulation at various points throughout the book; my goal here is that they provide a helpful backdrop against which to consider the ethical arguments that bear on the issue of "designer" children.

Genes and Genetics: Shaping the Human Body

Gene Structure

According to modern science, the basic physiological unit by which human heredity is governed is called a *gene*. Genes control the differentiation of the roughly fifty trillion cells of the human body, telling these cells what functions they are to perform, and when. Hence, from the beginning of life genes, in a sense, provide operating instructions to the cells in which they reside. In this way they ultimately command various traits of each individual human being: whether a person is tall or short; has brown, green, or blue eyes; has a round or a pointed nose; and much, much more. The human genome — the "unique genetic blueprint for each person" — consists of roughly thirty thousand genes located within the nucleus of each cell of the body.[2]

Physically, genes are comprised of DNA (deoxyribonucleic acid), long molecules wrapped around each other in double-strand fashion. The outside of this "double helix" is actually a phosphate-sugar backbone, while on the inside, molecules called nitrogenous *bases* are strung along in pairs. Hence, the whole structure is somewhat like a twisted zipper, the interlocking teeth made up of base pairs. These bases are strung along in specific order, only a small fraction of which comprises genetic information. Other sequences serve supportive functions, and still other portions of the DNA have functions unknown to us.[3]

DNA in the human being is wound up tightly around proteins and formed into *chromosomes*, which are found in the center (nucleus) of each cell. Hence, genetic information in the human being is located on these chromosomes, which come in matched pairs — twenty-two of them, plus two sex chromosomes (XX for females, XY for males), for a total of forty-six. Each somatic (nonreproductive) cell contains a full set of chromosomes, while the germ (reproductive) cells contain twenty-three chromosomes, containing only a portion of the total genetic material.

In human reproduction two germ cells, each containing twenty-three chromosomes, unite to form a zygote with forty-six chromosomes. Because most chromosomes are paired, each human being has two versions of most genes — half contributed by the mother, and half by the father. The process by which particular genes are ultimately passed on is somewhat random; hence, a person may or may not pass on a specific version of a gene to his or her progeny.

Genetic Expression and Disease

Ordinarily, genes function to create a harmonious whole in the human being. They direct the cell to produce amino acids, which make up proteins, in a process known as gene *expression*. That is, specific sequences of bases in a cell's DNA prescribe specific amino acids that the cell is to manufacture, and these amino acids in turn make up specific proteins. Hence, genes control when and how much of a protein is made for any given type of cell or tissue at any given time. In this way, the gene is "expressed" in the cell's functioning and, ultimately, in the attributes of the organism as a whole.

In most cases this extraordinary system results in the healthy differentiation, growth, and repair of all the cells of the human body. It should be stressed, however, that this system, though elegant, is far from static. The human genome is not unchanging; and when something changes (mutates) in a gene, a corresponding change is brought about in the protein produced and very often in the discernible characteristics of the organism itself. Moreover, if the mutation occurs in a germ cell, it will be passed on to the cells of the offspring.

Such genetic mutation is not wholly undesirable; in fact, it is thought to be responsible for the natural selection of organisms over long periods of time and thus for the process of evolution itself. However, the vast majority of genetic mutations are far from benign and can indeed lead to serious impairment in the way organisms function. Such harm is what we term genetic illness or disease.

By themselves, diseases that result from a single mutant gene and that are inherited in simple patterns ("Mendelian" diseases) number more than 8,500.[4] Diseases such as these are considered to be either *recessive* or *dominant.* In recessive disorders both versions of a particular gene (that contributed by the mother, and that by the father) must be affected for the disorder to be clinically manifested. Hence, someone can carry one copy of the errant gene, manifest no signs of the disease personally, and nevertheless pass on that one copy of the gene to his or her offspring. Only if both parents contribute an affected copy of the gene to their child will that child manifest signs of the disease. Cystic fibrosis is the most common example of a fatal recessive genetic disease in the United States today. Characterized clinically by viscous secretions of the pancreas and lungs, cystic fibrosis patients typically suffer from persistent coughing, wheezing, and potentially fatal infections. The disease strikes approximately one in 2,500 newborn Caucasians, although 4 percent of the Caucasian population carries the affected gene.[5]

In dominant disorders, on the other hand, only one version of the gene needs to be affected in order for a person to show clinical symptoms; hence, only one parent needs to contribute an errant gene in order for the child also to manifest the disorder. On average, in non-sex-linked dominant disorders, approximately half of all offspring of an affected parent will also be affected. Huntington's chorea, a degenerative neurological disorder characterized by abnormal movements and progressive dementia, is an example of a dominant genetic condition. Huntington's disease strikes about one in twenty thousand people.[6]

Not all genetic disease follows these patterns, however. There are also chromosomal disorders, where entire chromosomes may be wrongly added or deleted from a person's genome; Down syndrome is one such disorder where an extra copy of a particular chromosome (chromosome 21) is present. In addition, there are multifactorial conditions, where many genes interact with environmental conditions to create a disease; heart disease is one example. Moreover, some genetic diseases are not transmitted through germ cells at all, but rather are limited to specific somatic cells; certain types of cancer fit into this category.[7] Finally, it should be noted that it is a serious mistake to think that all human traits correspond with a particular gene; the vast majority of human characteristics, including most diseases, are the result of complex interaction between unknown numbers of genes and an organism's environment.

Human Intervention in Genetic Processes

Milestones in Human Genetics

Although the existence of what we now call human "genes" was posited decades earlier, it was not until the 1950s that the three-dimensional structure of DNA was more accurately determined. In the spring of 1953 Francis Crick and James Watson published their understanding of DNA as a "double helix"—the model that persists today. Another important milestone came in 1972, when scientists joined DNA fragments from two species, resulting in a deliberately created "recombinant" (sometimes called "genetically engineered") DNA molecule. Soon thereafter, recombinant DNA molecules were duplicated and grown in bacteria; substances such as human insulin and human growth hormone can be created this way. Safety concerns arose quickly, and in 1974 the Recombinant DNA Advisory Committee (RAC) was formed to advise the National Institutes of Health (NIH) on guidelines for research, which were first issued in 1976.[8] About the same time, the biotechnology industry began to blossom, based on these new developments. Genentech, established in 1976, was the first new firm specifically to apply recombinant DNA techniques to medicine. Since that time, hundreds of new firms have followed suit, and the industry itself has boomed.

One of the more visible uses of recombinant DNA techniques has been in the field of genetic screening and diagnosis. In 1982 these techniques were used to detect sickle-cell disease prenatally.[9] Of course, prenatal diagnosis makes use of a variety of technologies besides those related to recombinant DNA. Indeed, Ruth Schwartz Cowan holds that as early as 1949 the first fetal "condition" was diagnosed prenatally, when researchers determined the sex of cats on the basis of certain morphologic features of their nerve cells. Detection of other conditions soon followed, and by 1960 some physicians had begun to offer amniocentesis and therapeutic abortion to women who had a family history of hemophilia.[10]

Surely one of the most important and highly visible milestones in human genetic research is the Human Genome Project, the fifteen-year international effort to map and determine the chemical sequence of the entire human genome — all three billion base pairs. The Genome Project began to take shape in the mid-1980s, as techniques for sequencing human DNA began to improve. Although U.S. funding began earlier, the project's official starting date was October 1, 1991. It has been carried out at university and government laboratories throughout the United States and in conjunction with centers in England, Germany, Japan, France, and China. In addition, several other countries throughout the world maintain varying levels of involvement in the project. In the United States — the largest participant financially — the project is coordinated through both the Department of Energy (DOE) and the National Institutes of Health (NIH).[11]

The federal Human Genome Project, first slated for completion in 2005, was substantially urged on in its later years by the interest and involvement of private industry. In fact, a veritable race developed to completely decode the human genome. Companies such as Celera Genomics Corporation, Incyte Pharmaceuticals, and Human Genome Sciences, for example, privately invested huge efforts of their own, driven by the high profitability that access to (and patents on) portions of the genome promises. Driven primarily by the progress of Celera (the most visible competitor to the public project and led by the one-time NIH scientist Craig Ventner), the federal genome project completion date was pulled forward, first to 2003, and then, in "draft" form, to 2001. In June 2000 the leaders of the federal effort, on the one hand, and Celera's Ventner, on the other, announced jointly that each had essentially completed the process of sequencing the genome — though in fact portions of DNA remained unsequenced by both. Finally, in April 2003 the international consortium working on the project announced its successful completion.[12] Work continues to make use of the data for both research and commercial purposes.

The Human Genome Project has many potential benefits. Scientifically, it is expected to yield great insight into the process of human heredity, genetic mutation, and even our genetic relation to other species.[13] The most obvious benefit, however, is clinical: it could dramatically increase our insight into genetic disease and our ability to target and cure such diseases through genetic manipulation. In other words, as we begin to pinpoint the location on the genome of various disease-associated genes, the hope arises that eventually we will be more able to replace, modify, or repair "defective" gene sequences. In addition, some hold forth the possibility that drugs and treatments could be individually tailored so that they are well-suited to any given person's genome. In these ways we could make great strides in the scientific battle against a variety of devastating diseases, particularly those that are relatively less dependent on environmental factors.

Furthermore, if the Human Genome Project yields the kind of information that its strongest proponents hope for, there is no good reason to expect that the resulting clinical applications will be limited to curing human disease. That is, there certainly will be those who wish not only to cure or prevent human disease, but also to use genetic information, if possible, to deliberately select positive capabilities or characteristics of offspring — termed *enhancement* engineering. Legal theorist John Robertson, who has written extensively on matters of reproductive technology and genetics, comments that "the genome project will almost certainly accelerate a growing tendency of parents to choose or exercise control over offspring characteristics." In fact, it may go even further, so that, "in the distant future, engineering of offspring with specific characteristics, cloning, or even intentional diminishment of an otherwise 'normal' child may occur."[14] Although such interventions are admittedly still a distant prospect, the 1997 announcement of the first successful cloning experiment (of an adult sheep), as well as subsequent similar experiments, brought us one step closer to the prospect of full-fledged "designer children." Cloning is now debated with some regularity in both the mainstream and the scientific media, as are other forms of genetic manipulation once considered to be only remote possibilities.

Human Gene Therapy and Enhancement

Procedures for applying genetic technologies to cure serious genetic disease or to enhance human capabilities or characteristics are often lumped together under the term *human gene therapy.* Gene therapy describes the medical replacement or repair of "defective" genes in living human cells. At the present time, however, all that is technically feasible is the addition of "normal" genes to the DNA of individual patients who suffer from disease.

Such procedures are relatively recent. In 1984 the Recombinant DNA Advisory Committee created a new group, the Working Group on Human Gene Therapy (later the Human Gene Therapy Subcommittee), whose job was to review specific protocols for gene therapy. The first approved gene therapy procedure occurred in 1990, when researchers performed gene therapy on four-year-old Ashanti DeSilva. Ashanti was born with adenosine deaminase (ADA) deficiency, a life-threatening genetic disease that placed her at enormous risk of infection and required her near complete isolation in the sterile environment of her home. On September 14, 1990, researchers at the National Institutes of Health genetically modified Ashanti's own white blood cells and returned them to her bloodstream. The procedure is considered to be a partial success; although Ashanti will continue to require ongoing gene therapy treatments, she now can lead a relatively normal life, attending school and playing with other children.[15]

More recently, scientists in France announced in April 2000 that they succeeded in using gene therapy to save the lives of several infants suffering from a form of SCID (severe combined immune deficiency), an X-linked genetic disorder that decimates the immune system, similar to the disease suffered by Ashanti DeSilva. This more recent success initially was trumpeted as a scientific breakthrough because several technical obstacles encountered in earlier experiments were overcome. However, within three years two of those three children acquired leukemia-like illnesses, a development that has jolted the field of gene therapy and challenged scientists to find safer methods of implementation.

In spite of such setbacks, scientists tend to see great promise in gene therapy. In late 1995 one hundred clinical trials either had been approved by the Recombinant DNA Advisory Committee or were under review by the U.S. Food and Drug Administration. The majority of these (63 percent) were for various types of cancer, 12 percent were for HIV infection, and 22 percent were for genetic diseases of various kinds, including twelve procedures targeting cystic fibrosis. Gene therapy is thought to be most successful in attacking diseases that are caused by single-gene defects, and incurable, life-threatening diseases are more likely to be targeted. Besides ADA deficiency, other forms of SCID, and cystic fibrosis, the genetic diseases that have been targeted so far include Gaucher's disease, familial hypercholesterolemia, alpha 1-antitrypsin deficiency, Fanconi anemia, Hunter syndrome, chronic granulomatous disease, and purine nucleoside phosphorylase deficiency.[16]

One important distinction often made in discussions of human gene therapy is that between *disease therapy* and *enhancement.* This distinction, of course, is far from clear-cut. Indeed, it is no easy task to name exactly what we mean by *disease.* As many have pointed out, it is insufficient to identify disease merely as abnormality or difference, as there is nothing inherent in difference or variation that makes a particular biological, chemical, or mental state a disease. It may even be dangerous to equate difference with disease, since this could lead to viewing race, gender, or ethnicity as "diseases" of sorts. Moreover, many differences ordinarily are viewed as desirable or beneficial; for instance, we do not usually label those who are particularly smart or agile as diseased, although they do indeed differ from the norm. Bioethicist Arthur Caplan advocates that, for purposes of genetic intervention, disease should be understood not simply as equivalent to difference, but to abnormality *plus* dysfunction and disvaluation by an individual or group.[17]

Although the line between disease therapy and enhancement is sometimes a blurry one, most would agree that there is, nevertheless, a line to be drawn. An apt analogy is to liken the difference between genetic disease therapy and genetic enhancement engineering to that between talking and shouting; although the exact line between the two may not be identifiable, most people would agree that there is, in fact, a difference.[18] Indeed, making this line clearer is part of the aim of this book.

Another crucial distinction often made in the field of human gene therapy is that between *somatic cell* therapy and *germ-line* therapy. Somatic cell therapy refers to therapy on the ordinary cells of the body; germ-line therapy, by contrast, targets reproductive cells (or very early embryonic cells) and thus potentially affects not only an individual patient, but also that patient's descendants. Many supporters of somatic cell gene therapy — those who liken it to conventional medicine and thus find nothing ethically problematic about it — simultaneously reject germ-line therapy for extending the risks unacceptably far, into future generations and to people not even yet conceived.

The principal procedure used for gene therapy procedures today is *retroviral-mediated gene transfer.* In this procedure naturally occurring RNA viruses called *retroviruses* are engineered so that they can integrate into a strand of DNA without reproducing themselves and without destroying the host cell. These retroviruses are called "vectors," and they are used to add a "normal" gene to the host chromosome.

Numerous limitations in these current techniques of gene therapy exist. Most importantly, only random integration of retroviruses into the genome of each cell is possible at present; cleaner techniques, such as gene repair or replacement, are not yet feasible. Hence, dominant genetic disorders, where the presence of only one affected gene is manifested as a disease, are untreatable as of now. Moreover, germ-line gene therapy would require increased specificity of the site where the gene integrates into the host cell, so that the delicate environment of a developing germ cell, zygote, or embryo is not disrupted, and so that the modification to the cell endures throughout reproductive cell division.[19] This limitation presents perhaps the largest technical obstacle to germ-line gene therapy in human beings. Enhancement engineering would require an even higher level of technical sophistication, in order to coordinate the expression of the many genes that contribute to most physically observable traits. Finally, in all these cases the procedures involved are extremely expensive and require a high degree of expertise, which severely restricts the number of patients who can take advantage of them; until they become simpler and cheaper, they will not have a major impact on medicine and health care.

Despite the many technical difficulties, supporters of gene therapy remain optimistic. W. French Anderson, one of the most prominent scientists in the field and one of the designers of the first human gene therapy experiment, has even argued that the Human Genome Project may pave the way for gene therapy to be used not only to cure disease, but also to prevent disorders by providing protective genes before diseases become manifest. Anderson envisions that one day doctors will be able to inject vectors directly into patients the way that drugs are injected now. These vectors would target specific cell types, safely insert genetic information, and subsequently be regulated by normal physiological signals.[20]

Three Examples of Genetic Manipulation

Again, the only type of human gene therapy performed to date has been on somatic cells and has been aimed at curing serious disease. Nevertheless, it seems only a matter of time before other sorts of interventions follow. Indeed, the debate about whether germ-line therapy and enhancement engineering are ethical options has been raging for several decades, both in religious and nonreligious communities.

How do the three examples of genetic manipulation that we will consider here — genetic manipulation for the prevention of cystic fibrosis, for the enhancement of memory, and for sex preselection — fit into this overall picture of human gene therapy? Only the first (genetic manipulation for the prevention of cystic fibrosis) is technically an instance of human gene therapy per se. Still, each example represents a possible effort to alter the genome of a (future) child according to parental preference. Let us briefly examine each case.

Prevention of Cystic Fibrosis

Cystic fibrosis (CF) is a recessive single-gene disorder most often found among white persons of European ancestry. Among this population it is the most common genetic disorder. Because of a defective gene, the mucus-producing cells in a CF patient are unable to access sufficient water; thus they produce an abnormally thick mucus in the lungs and pancreas, making breathing and digestion difficult and leading to life-threatening bacterial infections. Patients with CF tend to have a persistent cough, wheezing, or pneumonia, and often they have trouble gaining weight despite excessive appetite. Treatment for CF depends on the stage of the disease, but one common means of treatment requires vigorous drumming on the back and chest to dislodge the thick mucus from the lungs. CF patients also must take antibiotics frequently to combat infection. Their median life expectancy is 33.4 years.[21]

Gene therapy does seem to hold great promise in the treatment of CF. In 1989 scientists discovered the defective gene that causes CF. Soon thereafter, in 1990, researchers successfully corrected CF cells in vitro by adding normal copies of the gene. The first experimental gene therapy treatments were administered in 1993, in which defective CF cells appear to have been successfully corrected in several individuals. Several clinical studies are currently underway using gene therapy to treat CF, and to date more than 180 people in the United States have undergone experimental gene therapy treatment. Current techniques treat affected airway cells, which eventually die off; hence, repeated treatments are necessary. Scientists have yet to identify the "parent cells" that produce CF cells, but the hope is that finding and treating these parent cells eventually will make repeated treatments unnecessary, so that individuals with CF could truly be "cured."[22]

There are, of course, treatments for CF other than gene therapy. In fact, drug therapies have been successful enough that one might question the wisdom of pursuing the more costly alternative of gene therapy. Pulmozyme, the first new drug for CF in thirty years, was approved by the U.S. Food and Drug Administration in 1993. In 1997 another promising new drug for CF was approved, an aerosolized antibiotic called TOBI (tobramycin solution for inhalation). Several other drugs, including INS37217 and azithromycin, are currently in clinical trials for use against CF. Yet another way to treat CF is to transplant healthy lungs into CF patients. This final option, however, presents all the usual problems associated with major organ transplants, such as expense, organ scarcity, and rejection by the body's immune system. In addition, lung transplantation does little for the other organs in the body that are affected by CF.[23]

Although all efforts at gene therapy to treat CF so far have been aimed at somatic cells, germ-line gene therapy for CF is not such a far-off idea. In fact, one of the clear benefits of germ-line therapy would be that many different cell types in many different organs presumably would all be affected, since the progenitor itself (i.e., the gamete or early embryo) would be the object of the therapy. This certainly would be a boon in diseases like CF, which are manifested in many different organs.[24]

If we can postulate a spectrum running from disease treatment, on the one hand, through enhancement, on the other, it is clear that efforts to treat and/or prevent CF fall near the disease treatment end. Certainly it is not the case that CF is the most devastating of all genetic diseases, ruining all patients' lives thoroughly and completely. Nonetheless, it is the most common fatal genetic disease in the United States today, and despite a thirty-three-year median life expectancy for CF patients, few would categorize it as an acceptably "normal" state of health. It is precisely because it is difficult to deny the status of CF as a serious genetic disease that I have chosen it for examination in this book; in a sense, the prevention of CF is a most attractive candidate for genetic manipulation.

Enhancement of Memory

The second example of genetic manipulation is memory enhancement in one's (future) children. In their book on human gene therapy LeRoy Walters and Julie Gage Palmer rightly point out that "the ability to remember words, names, facts, and experiences is one thing many people might like to improve for themselves and their offspring."[25] This is due in part to the fact that memory is commonly understood to be an important component of intelligence in human beings; enhancement of memory would be one way to use the tools of genetic engineering to impart to one's children a mental "edge" in the world.

Human memory is thought to involve the transfer of chemicals from one brain cell to another, so that electrical impulses are passed along the nerve cells. Presumably, genetic manipulation that facilitated this transfer, by improving the sensitivity of the receptors on these nerve cells, increasing the number of receptors, or increasing the amount of transmitter chemicals, would enhance memory. Walters and Palmer think that there is basis for optimism in this regard; they write, "The striking success of human studies in which memory has been facilitated by the administration of drugs affecting . . . receptors suggests that there is great potential for human genetic memory enhancements." Indeed, one study in 1991 achieved memory enhancement in human subjects by using drugs that facilitated the brain's transfer of chemicals.[26] Moreover, reported discovery in 1991 of the gene that encodes certain receptors in the brain cells of rats suggests that a future genetic manipulation for memory enhancement is not out of the question.

As in the case of genetic manipulation to prevent CF, one could imagine either somatic-cell or germ-line gene transfers by which memory could be enhanced in offspring. Yet the case of memory enhancement differs in a clear way from that of preventing CF, since the latter is, by all reasonable estimates, a serious disease. Hence, memory enhancement more closely approaches what might be categorized as enhancement genetic engineering.

Of course, as we noted earlier, this distinction is not always an easy one to maintain. What about an individual, for instance, whose memory seems abnormally deficient? In that case would genetic treatment be considered "therapy" or "enhancement"? As many have pointed out, it is not a straightforward matter to draw such a line separating a "normal" condition from an "abnormal" or "deficient" one, and much depends on the social context in which the condition is embedded. Nevertheless, if there *is* a line to be drawn, somewhere, between disease therapy and enhancement, most reasonable people would agree that memory enhancement in a cognitively "normal" human being does not fall on the "disease therapy" side of that line.

Because genetic manipulation to improve memory would, in most cases, be a clear case of enhancement (versus disease therapy), it is a useful procedure to submit to an ethical lens, particularly when compared to genetic treatment for the prevention of CF. Despite the fact that few would consider an average or even a bad memory to be a "disease," few would deny that they would like to possess a better memory, or that a better memory would help them along in the world. Whether or not genetic manipulation is an appropriate way to achieve such an improvement remains to be seen.

Sex Preselection

Sex preselection is unlike the other two examples of genetic manipulation offered above, for an obvious reason: it does not involve the direct manipulation of genes, but rather relies on "manipulating" human chromosomes indirectly such that a particular combination (coding for either a male or a female) is dictated in a human embryo. Again, in the human body it is the twenty-third pair of chromosomes that determines gender; females possess two X chromosomes, while males possess one X and one Y chromosome. Whether an embryo inherits two Xs or an X and a Y is determined by the male gamete (the particular sperm that fertilizes the egg), which can be either X- or Y-bearing.

Current techniques for sex preselection[27] range from low-tech practices such as controlling the timing of intercourse or a woman's diet to high-tech approaches such as X- and Y-bearing sperm sorting by means of centrifuge, albumin separation (sorting sperm by making them pass through a viscous solution), or, most recently, DNA staining with fluorescent dye followed by ultraviolet laser separation. This last method, trademarked as the "MicroSort" technique, is, without a doubt, the most significant new development in sperm separation; and, although still experimental, it is the only one that is considered to engage in "real" science within the broader scientific community. Still other, less technical approaches persist in popular thought; one fascinating study theorized that the age differential between mother and father affected a child's sex.[28] Of all these methods, the separation of X- and Y-bearing sperm, with subsequent artificial insemination, holds the greatest promise as a reliable technique of sex preselection. Presumably, in time these techniques will allow women and men to determine easily, reliably, and before conception which gender a (future) child will be. Although no totally reliable means of doing this is yet available, it is not unthinkable that ultimately one will be attained.

It is difficult to place sex preselection into the categorization of gene "therapies." It is clear to most people that being of one or the other gender does not make one "diseased"; it also is an uncomfortable proposition to classify sex preselection as "enhancement," though certainly some would see it this way. What is important here is that sex preselection constitutes yet another way that parents could, in theory, "shape" their children genetically. Indeed, many consider sex selection to be yet another part of a continuum ending in full-fledged "designer children." Dr. Sherman Elias, director of the division of reproductive genetics at the University of Tennessee at Memphis, voices this fear: "Today it's the preference for gender. Tomorrow we're making designer kids."[29] Hence, while not (or at least not yet) technically an instance of gene therapy, sex preselection, along with genetic manipulations to prevent serious disease and to enhance memory, can be seen as part of the overall urge to control the genetic makeup of our offspring. Moreover, a worldwide preference for boys, and a North American preference for firstborn children to be boys, lead many to fear that sex preselection would most often boil down to a way to select against females, making it particularly interesting (and many would say troubling) from a feminist standpoint. For both these reasons, sex preselection makes a useful third example in the present analysis.

Shaping Our Offspring: Some Ethical Considerations

Genetic manipulation presents a relatively new and, to some, frightening technological frontier. It is highly controversial in part because its potential benefits and dangers are numerous and profound. Without merely resorting to an exhaustive list, I will attempt in this final portion of the chapter to highlight some of these key advantages and pitfalls, particularly as manifested in the three specific examples of genetic manipulation under consideration. Most of these issues will arise in later chapters of the book; here I present them in order to crystallize, up front, some of the central questions that genetic manipulation presents.

Suffering, Well-Being, and Reproductive Choice

Why would an individual or a family opt genetically to manipulate their offspring? Among the multitude of possible reasons, the most straightforward and obvious, one that hardly needs articulation, is that genetic manipulation has the potential to relieve a child's suffering. Particularly in the case of efforts to treat or prevent serious disease, it is difficult to see any substantive difference between the aims of gene therapy and those of traditional medicine: both seek to fight human illness. Few would honestly deny that the child with CF (or Tay Sachs disease, or SCID) suffers, or that the burden carried by that child's parents is heavy indeed. Genetic manipulation represents a promising new way to treat, and possibly even prevent, such suffering. Moreover, in the case of germline genetic manipulation, such suffering could be prevented, in theory, for future descendants — altering the gene pool permanently.

The case for the prevention of suffering becomes even stronger if medicine lacks alternatives for effective treatment of a particular disease, or if gene therapy represents the most effective alternative. This could very well be the case for germ-line gene therapy in the treatment of CF. Because the disease affects many different internal organs, it is difficult effectively to treat the body completely. In theory, however, germ-line gene therapy would change the DNA of every cell in the body, since the germ cells themselves would be altered; hence, many different organs could be "treated" simultaneously. If successful, such an approach would represent a vast improvement over present piecemeal efforts to treat the disease.

In some cases the prevention of serious disease, and the suffering associated with it, can also be accomplished by sex preselection. A few genetic disorders are carried on the X chromosome; because females have two copies of this chromosome, they may carry the defective gene on one, while bearing a second, nondefective copy. Males, on the other hand, have no such second copy functioning to protect them. Hence, males are much more likely to be affected by such X-linked diseases, which include Duchenne muscular dystrophy, hemophilia, and Lesch-Nyhan syndrome. If a prospective mother knew that she carried the gene for an X-linked disorder, sex preselection theoretically would allow her to have a daughter, who in all likelihood would not suffer from the disease. Again suffering would have been prevented.

Parents may, of course, want to do more than simply treat or prevent serious disease; they may in fact want to take positive steps to improve the overall quality of life of their children. Gene manipulation could be seen as one very unique way to do this. Suppose, for instance, a parent of average intelligence comes to realize that his or her child would have a significant advantage in the world with a genetically enhanced memory. Since by most accounts memory is one factor in overall intelligence, a better-than-average memory surely would give that child a mental "edge," partially compensating for merely average intelligence. Moreover, it can be argued, an improved ability to remember names, faces, numbers, and dates would bring with it an increased sense of satisfaction and a diminishment of frustration for the child — goods in themselves. It would seem, on the surface at least, that to manipulate genes in this way would be to promote a child's welfare.

Similarly in the case of sex preselection, it can be argued that a child's overall quality of life would improve. If a child is of the particular sex most desired by her or his parents, is it not the case that that child will *feel* more desirable? In the words of one reproductive specialist, "A child of the wanted sex would be, without a doubt, a desired child."[30] In this case, it is not only the quality of life of the parents that would, presumably, improve; it is also the quality of life of the children, who would not, by their sex alone, disappoint. Indeed, in the extreme case, female infanticide — a practice that now occurs with alarming regularity in some parts of the world — could be averted by preselecting for boys. However one may feel about preselecting against girl children, surely that is better than killing them once they are born.

Supporters often tout a third major benefit of technologies designed to manipulate offspring genetically: these technologies expand reproductive autonomy. Whether they desire to have both girls and boys or to have only girls with blue eyes, parents presumably would have more choice and control if genetic manipulation were safely available to them. If one considers parental choice in reproductive matters to have a positive value of its own, genetic manipulation is one way to extend that choice.

Matters of Safety

Along with the great hopes of genetic manipulation come great dangers, as its critics are quick to point out. Foremost among these are safety concerns. Most current techniques of gene manipulation are still highly experimental, and relatively little is known about the potential side effects of the methods used. For instance, many researchers, including those who support efforts at gene therapy, believe that there may be a risk posed by the nonspecific insertion of genes (via retroviral vectors), which currently is accepted practice in somatic cell gene therapy. Some have noted the possibility that the vector will integrate into the middle of a gene that is essential to cell functioning and thus will kill or seriously harm the cell.[31] Furthermore, the case of the French infants who developed cancer confirms nagging fears that nonspecific gene insertion could somehow trigger disease. Finally, the use of retroviruses in gene therapy is itself questionable, since unengineered retroviruses are far from benign; perhaps the most notorious of these is HIV, the virus responsible for AIDS. What if a domesticated retrovirus regains the harmful capacity to reproduce itself, causing infection in the organism? In spite of its promise, all of these safety considerations present serious hurdles for somatic cell gene therapy.

The safety issues multiply when we turn to germ-line gene therapy, the form of genetic manipulation most likely to lead to scenarios of full-fledged "designer children." In germ-line therapy, problems that occur when the vector inserts itself into the cell could lead to mutations that are compatible with life but severely challenge the health of the offspring. Furthermore, the added gene may integrate at an inappropriate location, leading to a (dominant) lethal condition in the developing organism. Moreover, because all fetal cells would be affected by germ-line gene therapy, greater precision is needed to ensure that the inserted gene is properly expressed in the organism as it grows and develops. Finally, an obvious and serious safety-related danger of germ-line gene therapy is that all unanticipated negative side effects are likely to be visited not only on the immediate offspring, but also on future descendants. As bioethicist Agneta Sutton summarizes, "The price to be paid for any mishaps would be high."[32]

In the case of sex preselection, numerous safety considerations again threaten both women and offspring. In the newest method of sex preselection, MicroSort, serious questions remain about the effects of fluorescent staining and ultraviolet laser separation on sperm, including the long-term effects on offspring resulting from this technique. Even those who run the MicroSort clinic admit that many more healthy births will need to be successfully achieved before they are willing to declare the technique safe for widespread use.[33] Apart from these safety concerns, there is the simple danger that preselection techniques are still far from reliable, particularly when used to preselect for boys.[34] Although few doubt that the reliability of sex preselection soon will improve, it is clear that current statistics fall well short of a guarantee.

If scientists developed new methods for sex preselection — for instance, a pill taken before intercourse to determine the sex of offspring — safety considerations could further rise in importance. In all likelihood the person most at risk, both from techniques themselves and from research paving the way to such techniques, is the conceiving woman. Indeed, the history of reproductive technologies generally reveals an ugly pattern whereby women's health has been put in jeopardy in various ways, ranging from greatly increased infertility and uterine perforation risks from use of the IUD, to infertility and cancer in daughters of women for whom DES (diethylstilbestrol) was prescribed in the 1940s through the 1970s.[35] One certainly might expect at least the possibility that women's health could also be threatened in some further way by new technologies designed to preselect the gender of offspring.

"Playing God"

One major — albeit less concrete — danger often associated with genetic manipulation is that by tampering with genes, we overstep appropriate human limitations — that is, we try to "play God." According to this argument, manipulating the genome, particularly by way of germline gene therapy, places too much control, over human individuals or over human evolution generally, into the hands of mere mortals. Theologian Paul Ramsey was fond of the rhetorical exhortation not to "play God." In his best-known work on the subject, Ramsey maintains that human beings must resist a "messianic faith" in science that discards the limits of biological and historical existence. There is, in his view, room for significant, but not unlimited, intervention in nature; there are many things that theoretically we *could* do — including "grand designs" of "positive eugenics" — but that we *ought not* do.[36]

Even while acknowledging a grain of truth in the exhortation not to "play God," some theologians reject the term as rhetorical and unhelpful. For instance, Richard McCormick maintains that the phrase does little to enlighten the analytical process necessary to shed ethical wisdom on genetic intervention.[37] Nevertheless, the concern remains in the minds of many that genetic manipulation may lead us to a modern form of hubris — that is, to an ambitious power whereby we forget the limits appropriate to human nature, whatever those limits may be.

Objectifying Children

A third major objection to genetic manipulation is that to manipulate offspring genetically is to treat them not as dignified human subjects worthy of respect, but rather as objects of parental whim. According to this view, the closer we inch toward "designer children," the more we are apt to commodify children inappropriately and view them primarily as objects of ownership — in other words, "a special kind of 'property.' "[38] It is easy to see how such views function as a red flag for those already suspicious of our tendency to treat children with less than the full respect that human beings deserve.

This objection will be treated at some length in later chapters. For now, it is sufficient to point out that, at a minimum, the motives of those who wish to shape their offspring genetically — that is, to "design" their children — must be questioned. Whether gene manipulation constitutes an objectification of these children or simply a high-tech effort to attend to their welfare remains to be seen, and may depend in part on the details of any specific situation. Nevertheless, it is wise to remain wary of any shift in attitude whereby children are viewed increasingly as items to be selected in a store or catalogue.

A related consideration sometimes raised about germ-line genetic manipulation is the concern that it may deny to future children their "right" to a genome free from artificial intervention, and, more broadly, that it may wrongly restrict their future choices. This fear, of course, can be related to the above objection that to tamper with the human genome is to "play God." By engaging in germ-line therapy, it is held, we essentially perform changes on the genetic makeup of persons not yet born and therefore unable to consent. According to this view, such changes are, by their very nature, a violation of informed consent and hence unethical. At heart, the caution here is that such actions will inappropriately narrow the options of a child as she or he grows up, closing off the "right to an open future."[39]

Certainly it is true that germ-line genetic intervention would change the genetic makeup of persons unable to give their consent. However, proponents of such therapies argue that any reasonable future person *would* consent to certain interventions — for instance, interventions designed to protect against serious disease.[40] Still, the objection importantly reminds us that the consequences of genetic manipulation are indeed far-reaching, and that the impact of any changes we make could be felt far into the future. Moreover, parental autonomy is not the only form of autonomy at stake here; the rights and needs of the affected children must be adequately taken into account.

Disappointed Parental Expectations

Related to the concern that genetic manipulation may inappropriately objectify or commodify children is the worry that the prospect of "designer children" may raise parental expectations of their children to a dangerous level. If a parent were to take the relatively complicated steps necessary to genetically engineer a child, we should indeed fear that he or she would build up abnormally high hopes for what that child would be like, and would be less able to cope when things went wrong. In the case of memory enhancement, for instance, it seems likely that parents who would choose to improve genetically the memories of their offspring would themselves be prone to deep disappointment if their children failed to live up to their high hopes. Similarly, in sex preselection, parents may harbor unrealistic expectations about what a son or a daughter would be like; these hopes would be sorely dashed if their sex-preselected child did not fulfill these stereotypes. What if the desired ballerina ends up preferring basketball to dance? Teresa Marteau, director of the Wellcome Psychology and Genetics Research Group in London, points out that the prospect of designing children in this way may even compromise the goals of parenting. She asks, "Do we want to encourage conditional parenting, the kind of parent who says, 'I will love you only if you're a boy or a girl?' [That idea] eats a tiny bit into our humanity."[41]

Again, whether or not genetic manipulation causes parental expectations to rise to a problematic degree may depend on the details of any given situation and on any given parent. Moreover, foolishly high parental expectations certainly will find their way into our society, with or without genetic manipulation. Nevertheless, such manipulation may exacerbate an already existing problem in ways that we would be wise to avoid; hence, we do well to keep this danger at the forefront of our thinking.

Harm to Women

A major pitfall of genetic manipulation that is particularly relevant to sex preselection is that it could compromise the welfare of women. This concern stems in part from evidence that in many societies a strong preference for sons exists. In extreme cases, this preference has led to the widespread abortion of female fetuses and even in some places to female infanticide, prompting the now well-known statistic that an estimated sixty to one hundred million women are "missing" from the world's population.[42] Moreover, ratios in some countries where sex selection is widely practiced are becoming heavily skewed. In India, for example, in 2001 there were only 933 women for every 1000 men; and in the province around Delhi the number drops to 821.[43] One can imagine that improved techniques of preconceptual sex selection will only skew these demographics further, at least in parts of the world where the preference for sons is strong.

Even in the United States and Western Europe, where the preference fore sons is less obvious, there appears to be a preference that firstborn children be male. According to social psychologist Roberta Steinbacher, studies have shown that about 60 percent of Americans prefer that their firstborn child be a son. Moreover, one study of those who said they would use sex selection showed that 81 percent of the women and 94 percent of the men preferred firstborn sons. Although some hold that these numbers appear to have fallen in recent years, few contest that a preference for firstborn sons still exists.[44]

The consequences of a skewed sex demographic are potentially multiple, although whether or not these consequences are likely to occur is a point of major contention. Among the more common concerns are the prospect that an imbalance in the numbers of women and men could aggravate violence in society; that it could lower the status of women generally; that it could exacerbate patriarchal control over women (particularly if they are more often second-born) and harm women psychologically; that it could increase prostitution and the exploitation of the natural environment; and that it could accentuate class differences or lead to more women in poverty. In each of these cases it may be difficult or even impossible categorically to predict that the negative consequence will occur as a result of sex selection. Still, it remains at least a possibility that a preference for sons, especially firstborn sons, could lead to a society that tends to give more power to males and in which proportionally more women live in poverty.[45]

Another objection is less concerned with concrete consequences: sex preselection is, according to some, *inherently* sexist. In other words, sex preselection, for boys or for girls, involves parents making the most basic judgment that the worth of a human being rests first and foremost on gender.[46] Accordingly, there are few or no scenarios whereby sex preselection respects the inherent worth of the child-to-be. To select for or against children based on gender is to mistreat those children in a most fundamental way, as well as to contribute to a harmful social tendency to value persons according to gender.

Whether or not the welfare of existent women is in danger from sex preselection is unclear. Nonetheless, the foregoing objections highlight that there are potentially some good reasons, from the point of view of women as a whole (including future women), to at least hesitate before uncritically accepting the practice of sex preselection. Minimally, we should be questioning the motives of parents who opt for this form of genetic manipulation. Does the choice signify an inappropriate understanding of children, a valuation of their worth based upon gender? Such an understanding would be troublesome indeed.

Other forms of genetic manipulation likewise may result in unintentional harm to women, individually and as a group. Some of these we have already touched on in the discussion of safety considerations. Additionally, feminists fear that women generally may suffer an overall loss of control over their bodies and indeed over the entire reproductive experience as it becomes increasingly fragmented by the intrusion of technology. If reproduction itself is treated more like a mechanical process (re-*production*), the argument goes, then children become the products of that process, and women are akin to machines on an assembly line. This could be experienced by women as highly dehumanizing: it could significantly deconstruct and reshape our social interpretation of reproduction, altering women's own experience of their reproductive role. Furthermore, women in general may come to lose a substantial degree of control over their own bodies (in the context of reproduction), and support networks for women could further diminish — networks that traditionally have surrounded the experiences of gestation and birth. These forms of harm to women may be less tangible than others, but still they are highly significant to those viewing the situation through a feminist lens.

Socioeconomic Stratification

In today's tight healthcare economy, access to medical services is a major problem for many. When over forty-one million people in the United States lack health insurance for even the most basic care, it is reasonable to expect that high-tech procedures such as gene manipulation will be reserved largely for the relatively well-to-do. At least as it is now practiced and envisioned, gene therapy is too expensive to be an option for most people — a fact that troubles even its most ardent supporters. Until major technical breakthroughs lower the cost of gene manipulation, we can expect that its benefits will accrue disproportionately to those with the considerable funds needed to pay for them. Moreover, insofar as money continues to be spent on research and development for techniques of genetic manipulation, we can wonder about the justness of prioritizing these high-tech procedures while simultaneously failing to provide even a basic package of healthcare to everyone.

Such questions of justice in access to healthcare are a necessary part of any feminist and Christian inquiry into genetic manipulation. Above all, this is true because those who lack adequate healthcare are primarily, though not exclusively, the poor; and, the world over, the poor are predominantly female. A feminist and Christian ethical approach must ask, on some level, about the justice of spending vast sums of money on techniques that may in fact function to further marginalize poor women. This issue will appear at various points throughout this book as we consider who ultimately will benefit from techniques of genetic manipulation.

Threat to Diversity

Another concern that often arises in discussions of genetic manipulation is the possibility that it may lead to, or at least contribute to, a reduction in the diversity of the overall population. If children become heavily the product of parental design, it is argued, then short-term fashion could substantially influence how these designer children look, sound, and behave. Moreover, the ability to manipulate offspring genetically could lead us to "breed out" differences that prove difficult to deal with on a social level (such as disability), rather than challenge us to deal with them creatively.

As its supporters have repeatedly pointed out, it is extremely unlikely that the diversity of the population would be compromised in any serious way by techniques of gene manipulation; they simply do not affect enough individuals, and it is difficult to imagine that they ever would. A more serious problem is raised, however, by the possibility that techniques of genetic manipulation will allow society increasingly to disregard the need to deal creatively with difference. This has been a major objection on the part of some members of the disabled community who hold that genetic manipulation *in principle* constitutes a threat to the social well-being of disabled persons.

This issue, though not the central focus of this book, necessarily will arise in the context of feminist and Christian concerns to attend constructively to difference and to honor it as it appears in children (and other members of the human community). A feminist vision of community must affirm an inclusive welcoming of difference; to the degree that genetic manipulation poses a threat to this attitude, we should question its rightness.

Misuse by Dictators and Brave New World *Scenarios*

The final ethical concern to be raised here is the fear that genetic manipulation eventually will lead us to social structures à la Aldous Huxley's *Brave New World,* where society genetically engineers persons to fit into predefined social roles and castes. There are, of course, multiple variations on this theme in the public sphere, but all seem to boil down to some version of the idea that unscrupulous dictators could arise who will misuse genetic technologies to create a strongly class-based society buttressed by genetic design. Genetic technologies as they currently exist do not, of course, offer the possibility of such elaborate social consequences; however, genetic manipulation, particularly germ-line manipulation, may be seen as the first step on a slippery slope leading ultimately to such dismal social scenarios.

Most supporters of gene therapy quickly reject such concerns, holding that the best way to prevent the misuse by dictators of *any* technology is to foster and support democratic institutions. Despite the truth of this belief, anyone born in the late twentieth century cannot afford to dismiss out of hand the idea that genetic technologies could become attractive tools for powerful dictators; the racial hygiene movement in Germany in the 1930s and 1940s should have disabused us of any such cavalier attitude. Moreover, even if no deliberate, carefully constructed master social plan existed for the misuse of genetic manipulation, it is not unthinkable that even democratic social structures may participate in ill-advised eugenic policies; the history of the U.S. eugenics movement offers proof, as I show in chapter 2. So, although the extreme forms of these sorts of fears do seem rather alarmist, we do well to keep sight of history, especially recent history, and to guard against repeating its mistakes in the arena of genetic manipulation. The second chapter of this book is designed in part to provide some of this history in hopes of setting a context in which to evaluate genetic manipulation.

Approaching the Problem of "Designer Children"

"Designing children," it seems, is no easy ethical matter. Although the benefits of genetic manipulation are attractive, particularly in a culture such as that of the United States, where choice is a highly prized value, the dangers associated with it, from an ethical standpoint, appear to be real and multiple. Moreover, objections based on these dangers emerge from virtually all sectors of society, from the most conservative religious voices cautioning against a tendency to overstep human limitations, to the most radical activists arguing that genetic manipulation disrespects disabled persons and entrenches culturally constructed images of what is normal. No easy matter, indeed.

The aim of this book is not to exhaustively adjudicate all of these issues or points of view. Instead, I wish to focus on many of the foregoing ethical issues as they arise in the context of strong liberal, feminist, and Christian analyses of genetic manipulation. Necessarily, key concerns will move to the fore of the discussion, including the potential that genetic manipulation could harm the well-being of both the children to be "designed" and the women who bear them (or, indeed, all women in our society). Other concerns, by no means receding in importance, will come to light only secondarily. Importantly, the discussion will focus specifically on how the wisdom of feminist thought and of the Christian tradition can illuminate and help to fill out a norm of human flourishing, so that this norm may serve both as a corrective to a purely liberal analysis and as a guide for how we might more effectively approach the subject of genetic manipulation.

Before we turn to these various strands of thought for insight, however, it is important to do two things. First, any discussion of genetics in the wake of twentieth-century America is inadequate insofar as it fails to set itself into historical context. Hence, the next chapter is an attempt to examine a few key historical and social realities essential to informed deliberation. Second, because public discourse on the subject, particularly in the United States, has tended to revolve around the concept of procreative liberty, I spend the first part of chapter 3 examining a classically liberal approach to procreative liberty as it comes to bear on genetic manipulation. It is against this strongly liberal background, I believe, that the wiser insights of feminism (examined in chapter 3) and Christianity (chapter 4) are most powerful, and also have the most to say about the ethics of "designer children."

Notes

1. George J. Annas and Sherman Elias, eds., *Gene Mapping: Using Law and Ethics as Guides* (New York: Oxford University Press, 1992), 4.

2. LeRoy Walters and Julie Gage Palmer, *The Ethics of Human Gene Therapy* (New York: Oxford University Press, 1997), 4. Until very recently, the number of genes comprising the human genome was widely estimated to be closer to one hundred thousand. In February 2001, however, the publication of the first interpretations of the human genome sequence revised this long-held estimate. The figure is still somewhat disputed. The lower estimate of thirty thousand for the aggregate number of human genes, especially when compared with the genomes of other, simpler organisms, is particularly significant because it could indicate a weaker role for genes (relative to environment) in determining human biology. See Nicholas Wade, "Reports on Human Genome Challenge Long-Held Beliefs," *New York Times,* February 12, 2001, A1; Andrew Pollack, "Double Helix With a Twist," *New York Times,* February 13, 2001, C1.

3. Walters and Palmer, *Ethics of Human Gene Therapy,* 5.

4. Victor A. McKusick, *Mendelian Inheritance in Man: A Catalog of Human Genes and Genetic Disorders,* 12th ed. (Baltimore: Johns Hopkins University Press, 1998), 1:xvii.

5. Thomas D. Gelehrter and Francis S. Collins, *Principles of Medical Genetics* (Baltimore: Williams & Wilkins, 1990), 212–17.

6. Ibid., 208.

7. Walters and Palmer, *Ethics of Human Gene Therapy,* 14.

8. Office of Technology Assessment, Congress of the United States, *Human Gene Therapy: Background Paper* (Washington, D.C.: Office of Technology Assessment, 1984), 3.

9. Ibid.

10. Ruth Schwartz Cowan, "Genetic Technology and Reproductive Choice: An Ethics for Autonomy," in *The Code of Codes: Scientific and Social Issues in the Human Genome Project,* ed. Daniel J. Kevles and Leroy Hood (Cambridge, Mass.: Harvard University Press, 1992), 249, 253.

11. Michael D. Lemonick and Dick Thompson, "Racing to Map Our DNA," *Time*, January 11, 1999, 46; National Reference Center for Bioethics Literature, "The Human Genome Project," *Scope Note* 17 (Washington, D.C.: Kennedy Institute of Ethics, Georgetown University, 1999): 2.

12. See Paul Jacobs and Peter G. Gosselin, "An Unfolding Gene Map at 'Finish Line,' " *Los Angeles Times*, May 7, 2000, A1, A10; Lemonick and Thompson, "Racing to Map Our DNA," 46; National Human Genome Research Institute, "International Consortium Completes Human Genome Project," accessed at www.genome.gov/11006929.

13. David Suzuki and Peter Knudtson, *Genethics: The Ethics of Engineering Life*, rev. ed. (Cambridge, Mass.: Harvard University Press, 1990), 319.

14. John A. Robertson, "Genetic Selection of Offspring Characteristics," *Boston University Law Review* 76, no. 3 (1996): 422.

15. Larry Thompson, "The First Kids with New Genes," *Time*, June 7, 1993, 50–53; W. French Anderson, "The Best of Times, the Worst of Times," *Science* 288, no. 5466 (2000): 627–29.

16. Walters and Palmer, *Ethics of Human Gene Therapy*, 25.

17. Arthur L. Caplan, "If Gene Therapy Is the Cure, What Is the Disease?" in *Gene Mapping: Using Law and Ethics as Guides*, ed. George J. Annas and Sherman Elias (New York: Oxford University Press, 1992), 131–34.

18. Agneta Sutton, "The New Genetics: Facts, Fictions and Fears," *Linacre Quarterly* 62, no. 3 (1995): 86.

19. Walters and Palmer, *Ethics of Human Gene Therapy*, 67–68.

20. W. French Anderson, "Human Gene Therapy," *Science* 256, no. 5058 (1992): 666.

21. Cystic Fibrosis Foundation, "What Is CF?" accessed at www.cff.org.

22. Cystic Fibrosis Foundation, "Gene Therapy and CF," accessed at www.cff.org.

23. Cystic Fibrosis Foundation, "Progress in CF Research," accessed at www.cff.org.; Walters and Palmer, *Ethics of Human Gene Therapy*, 37; Cystic Fibrosis Foundation, *Lung Transplantation* (Bethesda, Md.: Cystic Fibrosis Foundation, 1999).

24. Walters and Palmer, *Ethics of Human Gene Therapy*, 62.

25. Ibid., 104.

26. Ibid.

27. I will not address forms of sex selection that occur after a child's (or future child's) sex has already been determined by natural processes — for example, amniocentesis with selective abortion or postnatal infanticide. Although these practices are excellent candidates for ethical analysis, they raise significantly different issues from those involved in sex preselection (i.e., the practice of choosing a child's sex prospectively).

28. In this study, conducted in England, it appeared that when a husband is at least five years older than a wife, their firstborn child is twice as likely to be a son; on the other hand, when wives are older than their husbands, they are twice as likely to have a daughter. See Brigid Schulte, "Want a Boy? An Age Gap Could Help," *San Jose Mercury News*, September 25, 1997, 6A.

29. Quoted in Nora Frenkiel, " 'Family Planning': Baby Boy or Girl?" *New York Times*, November 11, 1993, C6.

30. J. Egozcue, "Sex Selection: Why Not?" *Human Reproduction* 8, no. 11 (1993): 1777.

31. Walters and Palmer, *Ethics of Human Gene Therapy*, 40.

32. Sutton, "New Genetics," 84. For a fuller discussion of these safety hazards see Walters and Palmer, *Ethics of Human Gene Therapy*, 67–70.

33. Lisa Belkin, "Getting the Girl," *New York Times Magazine*, July 25, 1999, 26.

34. Although the practitioners of MicroSort now claim an 88 percent success rate for isolating X-bearing chromosomes, the rate for Y-bearing chromosomes is substantially lower (73 percent). Of pregnancies achieved by MicroSort in the initial study, 93 percent of the offspring were of the desired female gender. See E. F. Fugger et al., "Births of Normal Daughters After MicroSort Sperm Separation and Intrauterine Insemination, In-Vitro Fertilization, or Intracytoplasmic Sperm Injection," *Human Reproduction* 13, no. 9 (1998): 2367–70. In at least one case, a fetus of the undesired sex (female) was aborted by the conceiving parents. See Gina Kolata, "Researchers Report Success in Method to Pick Baby's Sex," *New York Times*, September 9, 1998, A1, A20.

35. Gena Corea, *The Mother Machine: Reproductive Technologies from Artificial Insemination to Artificial Wombs* (New York: Harper & Row, 1985), 148.

36. Paul Ramsey, *Fabricated Man: The Ethics of Genetic Control* (New Haven: Yale University Press, 1970), 149–51.

37. Richard A. McCormick, S.J., "Therapy or Tampering: The Ethics of Reproductive Technology and the Development of Doctrine," in *The Critical Calling: Reflections on Moral Dilemmas Since Vatican II* (Washington, D.C.: Georgetown University Press, 1989), 265.

38. Robertson, "Genetic Selection of Offspring Characteristics," 481.

39. Dena S. Davis, "Genetic Dilemmas and the Child's Right to an Open Future," *Rutgers Law Journal* 28, no. 3 (1997): 549–92. Davis founds her claims in this regard on Joel Feinberg's description of "rights in trust" held by children and "saved" until they are adults. Ultimately, such rights are based in the individual autonomy of the child.

40. Walters and Palmer, *Ethics of Human Gene Therapy*, 86.

41. Gail Vines, "The Hidden Cost of Sex Selection," *New Scientist* 138, no. 1871 (1993): 13.

42. Amartya Sen, "More Than 100 Million Women Are Missing," *New York Review of Books*, December 20, 1990, 61–66.

43. "Census of India 2001: Provisional Population Totals," at www.cyberjournalist.org.in/census/.

44. Roberta Steinbacher, "Should Parents Be Prohibited from Choosing the Sex of Their Child? Yes," *Health* 8, no. 2 (1994): 24. Interestingly, the limited data we have for the MicroSort technique indicates a preference for choosing girls. This, of course, may be due to the fact that MicroSort's "success" rate for girls is far higher than it is for boys. Moreover, in order to qualify for MicroSort, a couple must already have at least one child; hence, those seeking a *firstborn* male are automatically eliminated. The evident preference for girls among those seeking MicroSort stands in some contrast to the data from earlier franchised sex-selection clinics in the United States, Europe, and Asia, where, as of 1993, 236 couples had chosen to have boys, while only 15 had chosen girls. Unfortunately, this statistic is not further broken down into specific countries. See T. M. Marteau, "Sex Selection: 'The Rights of Man' or the Thin Edge of a Eugenic

Wedge?" *British Medical Journal* 306, no. 6894 (1993): 1704. At one sex-selection clinic in Hong Kong more than 90 percent of the clients choose boys. See Mark Landler, "Clinic Caters to Couples Seeking 'Precious Gem,'" *New York Times,* July 1, 2000, A4. On the MicroSort technique see Belkin, "Getting the Girl."

45. See, for example, Steinbacher, "Should Parents Be Prohibited?" 24; Dorothy C. Wertz, "Reproductive Technologies: Sex Selection," in *Encyclopedia of Bioethics,* ed. Warren Thomas Reich, rev. ed. (New York: Simon & Schuster Macmillan, 1995), 2215; Dorothy C. Wertz and John C. Fletcher, "Fatal Knowledge? Prenatal Diagnosis and Sex Selection," *Hastings Center Report* 19 (May–June 1989): 23–24. For a more skeptical view and a detailed description of these various potential negative consequences of sex selection see Mary Ann Warren, *Gendercide: The Implications of Sex Selection* (Totowa, N.J.: Rowman & Allanheld, 1985).

46. Tabitha M. Powledge, "Unnatural Selection: On Choosing Children's Sex," in *The Custom-Made Child? Women-Centered Perspectives,* ed. Helen B. Holmes, Betty B. Hoskins, and Michael Gross (Clifton, N.J.: Humana Press, 1981), 196.

Chapter Two

The Drive to Perfect Humanity

We stand in much greater danger from the well-wishers of mankind, for folly is much harder to detect than wickedness. — LEON R. KASS[1]

AS WE HAVE SEEN, on the surface, at least, contemporary efforts to "improve" the human condition by way of genetic manipulation can reflect quite reasonable and even noble intentions: the relief of suffering, the improvement of our children's lives, the advancement of our dreams for a world less filled with pain. Indeed, one can argue that there is very little difference between the highly technical step of genetic manipulation and the less technical measures that human beings have always tried to take in order to better the lives of our children: the provision of adequate nutrition, healthcare, educational or vocational training, and so on. However, a deeper exploration of the historical and social context of genetic manipulation complicates the picture, for there are distinct trends, both in contemporary U.S. culture and in recent history, that should cause us to pause before uncritically accepting genetic manipulation as a simple extension of our more ordinary efforts to help our children.

In the present chapter I examine two of these sociohistorical trends. First, within the context of the contemporary U.S. consumer culture, there is, I contend, a questionable and worrisome tendency to view children with a perfectionist eye — that is, as "products" of conception to be improved upon and eventually to be perfected. Second, reaching further (albeit not much further) back in time, we encounter the even more troubling phenomenon of explicitly eugenic thought, and in some cases the massive human atrocities that have accompanied such thought. Here I attempt to sketch the broad outlines of the history of this thought and to highlight the ways in which contemporary genetic manipulation does, and does not, resemble past eugenic efforts.

Both of these phenomena, it seems to me, are essential background to a fuller understanding of genetic manipulation, and both represent, at least in some part, well-intentioned efforts to "shape" our children and our society in a constructive direction. Certainly it would be wrong to jump too quickly to the conclusion that genetic manipulation must be abandoned altogether because of its connection with these more troublesome tendencies. Indeed, the danger in postulating these "worst-case scenarios" is that such a move can cause us to overlook the very important ways that genetic manipulation *is* different from past eugenic efforts, as well as to miss the distinctly positive benefits that genetic manipulation may have to offer. On the other hand, to fail to take account of this wider context is effectively to close our collective eyes to the ways in which we may be prone to repeating or perpetuating, unwittingly, some of our more insidious errors, individually and societally. The present chapter will provide some of this context so that we may more adequately formulate a responsible and thorough approach to present-day forms of genetic manipulation.

Contemporary U.S. Culture and the "Perfect" Child

One of the more disturbing trends that may be witnessed in at least some segments of contemporary U.S. social culture has to do with an increasingly unhealthy and even dangerous perfectionism that is focused on the lives of our children. Popular lore is replete with stories of children who grow into troubled adults because they experience unrelenting parental pressures during their childhood years. Furthermore, teenage suicide is commonly correlated with demands on children to excel at the expense of all else. Yet today, perhaps more than ever before, many of us (particularly, I suspect, many of us from well-educated, upper-middle social classes) seem compelled unquestioningly to pressure our children to achieve more and more, both physically and intellectually.

This tendency is particularly alarming because children are, arguably, the members of society least able to protect themselves against the harm inflicted by unrealistically high expectations.

Educational theorist David Elkind, in his study of "hurried" children, argues that many children today are encouraged by parents, peers, and society at large, including the media, to grow up too fast, to take on the physical, psychological, and social trappings of adulthood before they are prepared to deal with them. We in the United States dress our children as little adults; we hurry them into high-pressure summer camps and organized competitive sports; we apply intense pressure on them to "keep up" in school according to impersonal standardized tests. Elkind warns that this can lead to free-floating anxiety, "Type A" demeanor, school burnout, personality disorders, and various forms of negative behavior, including, in the extreme case, teen suicide, and that it often produces stress-related problems in adults.[2] In fact, Elkind asserts, pressuring a child to achieve too much too soon paradoxically can stunt a child's learning process in the long run.

Philosopher Nancy Ann Davis also holds that serious problems can result from contemporary pressures on children to "get ahead." Practices such as enrollment in high-pressure preschools and parental insistence on athletic prowess can, in her view, compromise a child's well-being, just as they in fact contradict the ideal of a parental love, which is unconditional and unselfish.[3] Moreover, Davis describes how the typically U.S. view of the state as being only minimally responsible for children's welfare encourages parents to view their children as private investments, whereby they should do everything they can to have the "best" child possible in order to justify the expense of having that child in the first place. Too often this means that children's true well-being is compromised by parental concern to have a "high quality" child, one who above all else fulfills parental needs, desires, and expectations. Ultimately, these attitudes reveal distortions in our understanding of who our children *are,* eclipsing their intrinsic worth.

As reproductive technologies have become increasingly sophisticated at predicting genetic and chromosomal abnormalities prenatally, this proclivity to demand high achievement from children has broadened to include a tendency to expect more "perfect" babies even from birth. Indeed, the increasingly accepted practice of aborting fetuses discovered to have genetic abnormalities (such as trisomy 21, indicating Down syndrome) attests to these elevated expectations.[4] Extrapolating one step further, some have envisioned a "perfect child syndrome," whereby couples might attempt repeated pregnancies, terminating all but the best test-passers.[5] We can even see signs of current perfectionist expectations in the marked rise in malpractice suits against obstetricians in recent years; it seems that we as a society are eager to find *someone* to blame when babies are born with any characteristic deviating from the "normal."[6]

Techniques of genetic manipulation can only exacerbate these trends. Parents who make use of reproductive technologies now will have powerful new tools that are sure to raise any unrealistic and potentially harmful expectations that they may have for their children. Moreover, the problem surely will increase as genetic technologies advance to where positive manipulations are routinely possible. If more and more overzealous parents make use of genetic techniques in order to manipulate their children-to-be, our definition of "normal" children will subtly shift, so that what is normal today may be less than acceptable tomorrow.[7] Furthermore, as parental expectations change to accommodate the new technologies, what once seemed merely a challenging characteristic with which to live (such as nearsightedness) may eventually become an unacceptable source of "misery" for both child and parent.

Even many advocates of genetic enhancement are quick to identify these attendant dangers. For instance, bioethicists LeRoy Walters and Julie Gage Palmer, who cautiously support some forms of enhancement genetic engineering, recognize the danger that perfectionist parents might use the new technologies to push their children to extremes, in a "new form of child abuse." Similarly, philosopher Glenn McGee, who also endorses certain forms of genetic manipulation in children, is nevertheless wary of the ways that these can create destructive parental expectations. Although he argues that genetic enhancement is, in theory, no more morally problematic than the use of piano lessons, private schools, or megavitamins, he admits that the attendant parental hopes that are raised can have a negative side: they can be unrealistic, misplaced, or lacking in foresight, ultimately restricting a child's horizons and setting oppressive standards that children are forced to meet.[8] Again, it is not that these technologies introduce new dangers, for the tendency to push children will exist with or without genetic manipulation; rather, technologies of genetic manipulation threaten to provide a new and potentially powerful outlet for our present destructive tendencies toward children.

All of this, of course, dovetails with a dramatic increase over the last thirty years in the human ability to control the reproductive process. The development and wide accessibility of the birth control pill and the legalization of medically assisted abortion have meant that couples have a high degree of control over whether and when they procreate. It can only be expected that many couples today might desire commensurate control over the *kind* of children that women bear. While applauding reproductive freedom on one level, we might also rightly fear that such an intense desire for control could ultimately cause us to lose sight of our essentially finite and vulnerable nature, for in the end, we cannot perfectly control our offspring.[9]

It is important to recognize that this drive to "perfect" our offspring exists for us today within a highly technological and consumerist U.S. society, where even our babies and children are subtly yet increasingly commodified. Oliver O'Donovan has incisively pointed out that a technological society tends to think of everything that it does as a kind of mechanical production, a project of pure human will.[10] In the United States today this is disturbingly the case with children, the "products" of conception, and, in the view of some, an appropriate object of "quality control." In fact, this is how Dr. Saul Lerner, a former chairperson of the American College of Obstetricians and Gynecologists' District I, referred to the drive to ensure the health of newborns by way of preconceptive counseling: "What we have to do now is concentrate on quality control. . . . If more babies are surviving, we've got to make sure they are better babies."[11] Such approaches highlight the growing tendency in our society to treat children a bit like consumer goods, valued increasingly for their quality and utility rather than simply in and of themselves. Put differently, we in contemporary U.S. society are prone to commodifying *everything,* even our children.

Some bioethicists have expressed serious reservations about the tendency to focus on "quality" in offspring. Agneta Sutton, for instance, warns that "when people start asking for babies with — or without — certain qualities, there is the risk . . . that the value of children will be measured in units of health and performance quality, social utility and parental satisfaction. That is to say, there is the risk that their intrinsic value and dignity as human beings, as our neighbors and fellow images of God will tend to be forgotten." Sutton goes on to say that our desire to enhance children genetically implies the refusal to accept children unconditionally, thereby degrading them and impoverishing ourselves.[12] Certainly many would disagree, arguing that the distinction is, at best, blurry between genetic enhancement and, for example, expensive private tutoring or even standard childhood immunizations against disease. Still, the cautious approach highlights a tendency that does seem particularly seductive in U.S. society today: viewing children purely as objects for manipulation (and "quality control") rather than as persons in their own right, intrinsically valuable and dignified just as they are. I will examine this theme in more detail in chapters following. Here it is sufficient to note that perfectionist tendencies toward children, and the accompanying proclivity toward children's objectification and even commodification, already seem to exist in U.S. society, and they do little to reassure us that the further development and accessibility of these technologies will protect and enhance the intrinsic dignity of children.

Finally, this entire discussion must be set responsibly into the context of an abysmal lack of social services for persons with disabilities in the United States today. The trend toward seeking more "perfect" children coincides with a societal tendency to shrug off responsibility for caring for disabled persons. Many parents simply do not feel equipped to care for the needs of "imperfect" children. Whether or not these parents are fully justified in their fears, the banner of "economic realism" surely has masked a growing social hard-heartedness toward the disabled and a desire to save financial resources at their expense. One former health-systems analyst in the office of the Surgeon General puts it bluntly: "If we allow our genetic problems to get out of hand...we as a society run the risk of overcommitting ourselves to the care and maintenance of a large population of mentally deficient patients at the expense of other urgent social problems."[13] Whatever the merits of "perfecting" our offspring genetically, we should rightly fear that it could become a reason to turn away from the less-than-perfect — that is, an excuse for refusing to invest social resources into bettering the lives of disabled persons.

Eugenic Thought in Western Society

The tendency toward perfectionism described here has a distinctly contemporary flavor, taking place as it does in an increasingly efficiency-oriented society in which we human beings have a great deal of technological control over our world in general. However, perfectionist thinking regarding our offspring certainly is not a new phenomenon. Until relatively recently, such thinking often took the form of explicitly eugenic thought. Eugenic ways of thinking have been around a long time; indeed, at least since Plato's *Republic* there has existed a significant strand of Western thought that has stressed selective human breeding as a means of benefiting individuals and, more commonly, society in general. In the late nineteenth and early twentieth centuries eugenic thought truly began to flourish in the Western world, leading, in the not-so-recent past, to some of the worst horrors that the world has ever witnessed.

Daniel J. Kevles begins the 1995 edition of his renowned study on the history of eugenics with a pointed remark: "The specter of eugenics hovers over virtually all contemporary developments in human genetics."[14] Indeed, one cannot begin to address the ethical implications of genetic manipulation without encountering head-on the fear that such manipulation inevitably leads us down a "slippery slope" to the eugenic practices (and associated atrocities) of the past. On the surface, at least, such fears are not unfounded, for many of the concerns that drive the development of genetic technologies today — for instance, the desire to eliminate deadly disease, or the wish to improve people's capability to function well in the world — also appeared as motivating forces in the Anglo-American eugenics movement of the late nineteenth and early twentieth centuries and in the racial hygiene movement in Nazi Germany. Yet, as we will see, the parallels between contemporary genetic science and historical eugenics are far from perfect, and we must resist the tendency to equate the two phenomena.

Although eugenic thought can be traced back at least to Plato, the term "eugenics" was coined in the late nineteenth century by its most well-known proponent, Victorian polymath Sir Francis Galton, cousin to famed evolutionary theorist Charles Darwin. "Eugenics" derives from a Greek word meaning "good in birth" or "noble in heredity." Galton intended the term to mean the "science" of improving human stock by giving the "more suitable races or strains of blood a better chance of prevailing speedily over the less suitable."[15]

Eugenic ends can, in theory, be achieved in a variety of ways; accordingly, the concept of eugenics is divisible into "positive" and "negative" eugenics. Positive eugenics refers to the effort to foster greater representation in society of people considered socially valuable — for example, by encouraging them to marry within their own ranks or to procreate more. Negative eugenics, on the other hand, denotes the effort to encourage the socially "unworthy" to procreate less or even to prevent them from procreating at all. This might include methods such as sterilization or marriage restriction laws, or even eugenically motivated restrictions on immigration to prevent "undesirables" from joining a particular society in the first place. Both positive and negative eugenics have been present in the movement's history.

Sir Francis Galton and the Seeds of Eugenics

Sir Francis Galton, usually considered the "father" of the eugenics movement, published his best-known work, *Hereditary Genius*, in 1869. There he argued that human ability may be carefully correlated with reputation, and, moreover, that such natural ability is primarily a product of inheritance. Some are born with significantly more talent and intelligence than others, and these are the people who are most socially valuable. By contrast, the "unfit" he considered to be primarily a burden to society. Hence, in his view, society should encourage the talented and the intelligent to propagate early and often; for "as it is easy . . . to obtain by careful selection a permanent breed of dogs or horses gifted with peculiar powers of running, or of doing anything else, so it would be quite practicable to produce a highly gifted race of men by judicious marriages during several consecutive generations."[16] Galton believed that each person has a tremendous obligation to society to act in a eugenically "wise" manner; to do less is tantamount to wishing ill on future persons. In other words, eugenics was, for Galton, a simple matter of duty.

The central goal of Galton's eugenics was for human beings to take charge of human evolution. As he once put it, "What Nature does blindly, slowly, and ruthlessly, man may do providently, quickly, and kindly."[17] Indeed, Galton viewed eugenics as a kind of religious obligation and a welcome substitute for orthodox religious doctrine. He was a skeptic of orthodox faith and considered himself to be first and foremost a scientist, even though he was largely untrained in the sort of research that he pursued.[18] Yet in eugenics it seems that he and many others found a new home for their eschatological hopes, and eugenics carried almost religious significance for many who envisioned a better society.[19]

Galton urgently felt that the very welfare of society depended on such eugenic improvement. In his view, civilization had developed to the point that its demands were not matched by the intelligence and abilities of the average member of his "race." To rectify the situation, Galton suggested a variety of eugenic measures over the course of his career, including state-sponsored competitive exams (with the winners encouraged to marry and procreate), and state rankings of individuals according to their ability (with more children authorized for those ranking higher on the talent-intelligence scale). Galton eventually gave up on the involuntary aspects of these programs, but he hoped to the end that the dissemination of eugenic ideas and theories of evolution would lead to voluntary eugenic marriage practices.

Galton's legacy in the field of eugenics was immense. His ideas gradually took root on both sides of the Atlantic, and in 1904 he established a Research Fellowship in National Eugenics at University College in London, and later a chair, the Galton Eugenics Professorship. Out of the former also grew the Galton Laboratory for National Eugenics. This laboratory became an internationally renowned academic center for the study of eugenics, and later of human genetics.

The Eugenics Movement in the United States

Eugenic thinking was by no means limited to England. After the turn of the century eugenics movements sprang up in many different countries around the globe, including, prominently, the United States, which soon became one of the world's great centers of eugenic thought and activity. Indeed, in the early 1900s eugenic thought became wildly popular in mainstream U.S. culture, and (as in England) eugenic groups and societies seemed to sprout up everywhere.

Despite this grassroots strength, however, the movement did have its leaders, and first among these was Charles Davenport. In 1910 Davenport, a biologist, founded the Eugenics Record Office in Cold Springs Harbor on Long Island. The office was set up to conduct research via house-to-house surveys and by studying records from prisons, almshouses, and institutions for the mentally deficient, deaf, blind, and insane. In addition, the Office supported scholarship students to study human heredity and collect data, primarily on the subject of "feeblemindedness," for analysis. Although the scientific dubiousness of its assumptions is now widely recognized, the Eugenics Record Office in Cold Springs Harbor was, at the time, without question the leading institution in the United States for eugenically oriented study and research.

Davenport's vision favored "good stock," particularly the white Protestant majority. Unlike Galton, he was primarily a negative eugenicist, and he supported a selective immigration policy and state-enforced sterilization. In the view of historian Kevles, Davenport was "greatly given to oversimplification and little to self-critical reflection." Moreover, not only was his vision based on bad science, but also it was cruel and offensive, expressing "in biological language the native white Protestant's hostility to immigrants and the conservative's bile over taxes and welfare."[20] Like the worst aspects of the movement that he helped spawn, Charles Davenport's "scientific" interests came to serve insidious race and class prejudices masquerading as the promotion of human welfare.

Harsh judgment now, however, does little to explain how eugenicists such as Davenport justified their views and why these views took hold of the public consciousness so widely. Indeed, one of the most noteworthy aspects of the eugenics movement is that its supporters were ardently convinced that human welfare depended largely on eugenic measures. They were concerned with the deterioration of intelligence in the population and were taken with the idea of eradicating social "defect" in society. Moreover, one is struck by the religious justifications commonly offered for these views. Many saw fit to meld eugenic ideas with Christian doctrine. For instance, Albert E. Wiggam, journalist, author, and lecturer, once described eugenics as "simply the projection of the Golden Rule down the stream of protoplasm. . . . Do unto both the born and the unborn as you would have both the born and the unborn do unto you." In a similar vein, Protestant sermons of the time held that the Bible was a eugenic book and that Jesus was born into a family representing "a long process of religious and moral selection."[21] Though by no means universal, such "religious" justification did hold a prominent place in eugenic thought.

A less overt justification for the explosion of eugenic thought in the early twentieth century was the onset of social changes that were straining the United States at the time. Industrialization and the increase of big business inevitably led to the growth of urban sprawl and associated problems such as prostitution, crime, alcoholism, and disease. New waves of immigration precipitated fierce competition for jobs and led to tides of xenophobia. Moreover, a surge in eugenic thought during the Great Depression leads one to speculate that tight budgets had more than a small role in spawning a public desire to "improve" the social makeup.

Eugenic Policies

Whatever the reasons, the first third of the twentieth century saw eugenic programs gain a strong foothold in the United States. Although some went so far as to suggest that mothers of babies with deformities should commit infanticide, most eugenic thought was channeled into more moderate public policies such as immigration curtailment, marriage restriction laws, and sterilization.

The impact of eugenic thought on the immigration restriction policies of the 1920s should not be underestimated. Eugenicists who stressed so-called genetically based racial differences argued that immigrants from eastern and southern Europe brought an "inferior" genetic makeup to the United States and therefore should be excluded. Race appears to have played a large role in the 1923 hearings of the House committee on Immigration and Naturalization; one Jewish member of Congress remarked in 1923, "If you had been a member of that committee you could not help but understand that they did not want anybody else in this country except the Nordics."[22] Indeed, the 1924 U.S. Immigration Act, which sharply reduced immigration into the United States, was structured so as to disproportionately affect immigration from eastern and southern Europe.

A second front on which the U.S. eugenic battle was waged was that of marriage restriction. In some cases this sort of approach took the more benign form of publicly encouraging voluntary "eugenic" thinking in the realm of marriage and family. For instance, throughout the 1920s "fitter family" contests took place at state fairs across the country, wherein contestants provided a detailed family history and all family members underwent medical and intelligence testing. The winners were rewarded with state trophies and were prominently celebrated in local newspapers. Stricter measures, however, included the marriage restriction laws that spread throughout the states. By 1914 thirty states had laws on their books restricting marriage of the "unfit." In many cases the laws were justified on the basis that "idiots" (with a supposed mental age of one or two), the insane, or even the "feeble-minded" (a catch-all category for those displaying any of a wide variety of mental deficiencies or even socially deviant behavior) were unable to enter into contracts or would make poor parents. Some laws, however, were justified specifically on eugenic grounds.[23]

Perhaps the most insidious of all eugenic efforts in the United States was the now well-known movement for involuntary sterilization. Relatively uncomplicated sterilization methods were developed around the turn of the century, giving a boost to the idea of sterilizing for eugenic purposes. The first state law to mandate sterilization based on eugenic principles came in 1907 in Indiana, and by the mid-1930s an estimated twenty thousand people had been forcibly sterilized in the United States. Although the zenith of involuntary sterilization came in the 1930s, some states continued well beyond that time, and by 1963 some sixty thousand persons in the United States had been sterilized pursuant to state laws.[24]

Harry Laughlin, superintendent of the Eugenics Record Office from 1910 to 1939, was infamous for his part in this sterilization movement. In 1922 he proposed a "model sterilization law" that became the prototype for many later laws, although few followed all of Laughlin's suggestions. According to this model law, those considered for sterilization should include the "blind, including those with seriously impaired vision; deaf, including those with seriously impaired hearing; and dependents, including orphans, ne'er-do-wells, the homeless, tramps, and paupers."[25] Although people placed in categories such as the "feeble-minded" and the "insane" commonly were the target of involuntary sterilization, it is noteworthy that here Laughlin openly advocated sterilizing people who were poor. Indeed, sociologist Mark Lappé points out that historically, sterilization programs have been directed at the poor "in the mistaken belief that they were the embodiment of defective genes."[26] Nowhere is this deplorable truth more clear than in the grievous case of Carrie Buck, described in the appendix. Buck's case provides a chilling example of the way eugenic thought was employed to trample on the rights of poor or otherwise socially marginalized people, directing society's attention away from their basic worth as human beings.

The Racial Hygiene Movement in Nazi Germany

The legacy of eugenic thought took its most atrocious form in Nazi Germany. We in the United States have a tendency to distance ourselves from Nazi beliefs and practices; after all, a war was fought and millions of lives lost in order to resist a Nazi victory. Yet, unbeknownst to most Americans, much of Nazi policy was founded on principles that took their impetus from the U.S. eugenics movement. Indeed, in 1923 Fritz Lenz, a German physician and later a leading ideologue for "racial hygiene" under the Nazis, berated his compatriots for their backwardness vis-à-vis their U.S. counterparts with regard to eugenic sterilization. In 1936 Harry Laughlin, head of the Eugenics Record Office, accepted an honorary doctorate in medicine from the University of Heidelberg; in his acceptance letter he declared that he viewed the award both as a personal honor and as "evidence of a common understanding of German and American scientists of the nature of eugenics."[27] It seems that there existed a sort of mutual admiration, and at times a sense of competition, between American eugenicists and their counterparts in the Nazi racial hygiene movement.

Like the eugenics movement in the United States, the racial hygiene movement subordinated individual rights to the greater good of the whole, in this case the German *Volk*. In fact, according to one prominent historian, the *Volk* became a sort of holy concept; in racial hygiene, "we may say that mysticism, especially communal mysticism, was given a biological and medical face."[28] If American eugenics can be considered idealistic, then, German racial hygiene took that sort of idealism to an extreme, warning against the ratio of births among the "fit" and the "unfit," and, ultimately, the danger of *Volkstod*—"death of the people." This nationalistic idealism also included an attack on "exaggerated" Christian compassion for the weak individual; such sentimentalism was seen as wrongly devaluing the health of the people as a whole. Christian charity and the "ill-conceived" love of neighbor were thus rejected as overly individualistic. According to German racial hygiene, the life of the individual was secondary to the aim of a hereditarily sound and racially pure *Volk*.

Importantly, physicians played a central role in the racial hygiene movement. Medical doctors were considered not just caretakers of the sick, but rather "cultivators of genes," "biological soldiers," and "physicians to the *Volk*." Their obligation to the people as a whole superseded their obligation to individuals. Moreover, physicians were urged to teach their patients that any right to their bodies was properly subordinated to their duty to be healthy. This sort of claim was seen as a reassertion of the moral high ground of medicine past, a "return to the ethics and high moral status of an earlier generation . . . which stood on [the] solid ground" of the Hippocratic oath.[29] It seems that biomedical ethics, at least as understood by racial hygienists, stood at the heart of the Nazi vision.

As in the United States, eugenic sterilization played a major role in Nazi policy, particularly in its earlier phases. Though patterned in part on U.S. sterilization laws, however, Nazi Germany's approach was much more dramatic and severe. In 1933 a sweeping law was passed authorizing compulsory sterilization for those with "hereditary" disability: feeble-mindedness, schizophrenia, manic-depression, epilepsy, Huntington's chorea, genetic deafness or blindness, severe drug or alcohol addiction, or physical deformities that interfered with locomotion or were "grossly offensive." No one knows for sure how many people were sterilized under this law, but the most reliable estimates seem to hover around four hundred thousand. Incredibly, there was relatively little public opposition to sterilization. Even the Roman Catholic Church in Germany opposed it only weakly, at least on an institutional level, and the Protestant Church there generally did not oppose Nazi sterilization laws.[30]

Sterilization was, of course, accompanied by other eugenic measures. These included marriage restriction laws that prohibited the espousal of persons of different "racial" backgrounds. Furthermore, the Nazis instituted generous loans and loan forgiveness programs for biologically "sound" couples whose fecundity was seen as fortifying the *Volk*. Even more nefarious was the criminal *Lebensborn* ("Spring of Life") program, involving the kidnapping of eugenically desirable children from Nazi-occupied territories and welfare assistance to SS families with "racially valuable" children.[31] Yet all of these practices pale in comparison to the mass murders that constituted later racial hygiene policy. In 1939 "mercy killings" began with the murder of deformed and retarded children, and very soon extended to all "incurably sick" and "mentally diseased or disabled" adults as well. Eventually, the "sick" came to include all Jews — and not only Jews, but also Gypsies, communists, homosexuals, and a wide variety of "antisocials" — regardless of the state of their physical or mental health. This line of thinking ultimately paved the way for the slaughter of some six million European Jews. Indeed, the choice to exterminate Jews by gassing them in concentration camps, in what came to be known as the "Final Solution," was due in part to the fact that the necessary technical apparatus already existed for the mass destruction of mental patients.[32]

Again, it is imperative to emphasize that these murders were largely planned and administered by medical professionals. For the most part it appears that doctors fulfilled their task voluntarily; they were not *ordered* to murder patients so much as they were *empowered* to do so by Hitler.[33] Furthermore, no clear dividing line existed in the Nazi mindset between the racially "inferior" and the mentally or physically "defective." Both constituted a threat to a racially "pure" Germany.

It is glaringly apparent that, in the case of Nazi Germany, there was indeed a "slippery slope" between eugenic attitudes and policies, on the one hand, and mass murder, on the other. Moreover, intermediating these two approaches were the physicians, putting biological science to work for the "good of the whole." For whatever reason — and one could speculate indefinitely — eugenic thought took root in Nazi Germany in a way that eventually helped pave the way for some of the greatest atrocities of the twentieth century.

The Demise of Eugenic Thought — and Its Reincarnations

Historian Philip Reilly calls the Nazi racial hygiene program "eugenics run amok." Yet, in his view, the initial decline in popularity of eugenic thought in the United States does not appear to be strongly connected with the revelation of Nazi horrors, though the latter most certainly contributed to it. Indeed, opposition to eugenic thought was growing in the United States long before the Nazis even rose to power. The Roman Catholic Church officially opposed eugenics in 1930, linking it with modern permissiveness and erotic passion that threatened the integrity of the family. Far earlier, however, the Church stressed that every human being, even those whom eugenicists considered biologically "unfit," deserved respect as a child of God.[34]

Nonreligious opposition to eugenics also played a key role in moderating its strength. For their part, nonreligious humanists began to resent the ever mounting authority of science that many of them saw embodied in eugenics. In the scientific world opposition to the "pop-science" approach associated with eugenics gradually led many scientists to distance themselves from the field, believing that eugenics was tarnishing the genetics enterprise. Moreover, as scientists learned more about the complexity of human heredity, it became harder to give credence to simplistic eugenic thinking. In 1940 the Eugenics Record Office finally was shut down after a blue-ribbon panel of scientists determined that its data were taken and analyzed using faulty methods.[35]

Still, vestiges of eugenic thought survived in the field that now is known as human genetics. For example, the beginnings of genetic counseling arose as early as the 1940s, and in 1974 a former analyst in the U.S. Surgeon General's office suggested a money-saving program of voluntary diagnosis and abortion for fetuses with Down syndrome.[36] In another example of revived eugenic thought, Arthur R. Jensen, a professor of education and psychology, wrote an article in 1969 that insisted on "the possible importance of genetic factors in racial and behavioral differences." He went on to couple so-called racial genetic differences with the possibility of dysgenic trends in urban slums, igniting anew the debate about race and intelligence. His work helped spur on the newly developing and highly controversial field of sociobiology.[37]

One of the more explicit "reincarnations" of eugenics in the United States in recent times is the Repository for Germinal Choice, founded in 1971 by Robert K. Graham, a millionaire industrialist. Graham, a political conservative, intended this sperm bank to aid in the overall genetic increase of intelligence; hence, he solicited exclusively the sperm donation of Nobel laureates and actively searched for healthy, intelligent female recipients. The Repository for Germinal Choice existed until very recently in Escondido, California, though it began accepting sperm donations not solely from Nobel laureates but from scientists generally.

Arguably, if eugenics were to surface in any widespread manner in the U.S. market economy, the most likely way would be on an individual basis, in the subtly eugenic choices that persons and couples make with regard to the traits of their offspring. Today, for instance, through the use of amniocentesis and selective abortion, families can choose against bearing a child with certain known diseases or disabilities, such as Down syndrome. Indeed, several screening tests in pregnancy for genetic disorders are now considered routine by most physicians. Historian Daniel Kevles speculates that in the future families could have greater choice and even more access to "improved" (e.g., more intelligent or athletic or better-looking) babies, maintaining that "a kind of private eugenics could arise from consumer demand."[38]

In a related vein, it can be argued that eugenic ends already are subtly incorporated into lists of diseases chosen as making a fetus "suitable" for selective abortion. Indeed, genetic screening, treatments, and therapies may lead to a kind of a "back door to eugenics," since they reflect a de facto acceptance of the policy of genetic exclusion and are often targeted at particular ethnic or cultural groups.[39] Moreover, while this subtle "back-door" eugenics may be the great danger in the United States, not-so-subtle forms of eugenics still persist elsewhere around the globe. For instance, in 1988 China's Gansu province adopted an explicitly eugenic law designed to "improve" the quality of the population by banning the marriage of mentally retarded people unless they are first sterilized.[40] Similarly, in Singapore in the 1980s a variety of measures were taken both to induce more well-educated women to procreate and to provide incentives for less well-educated (and poorer) women to be sterilized, on explicitly eugenic grounds. In 1983 Singapore's prime minister Lee Kuan Yew exhorted, "We must expend our limited and slender resources [on naturally superior individuals] in order that they will provide that yeast, that ferment, that catalyst in our society which alone will ensure that Singapore shall maintain its preeminent place in the societies that exist in South East Asia."[41] These examples may be the most egregious ones, but they are not isolated instances. Other explicitly eugenic policies can be found in India and parts of Latin America, and some suggest that negative eugenic intent even showed up in a 1988 proposal for a European human genome project put forth by the European Commission.[42]

Wherever they appear, eugenically oriented policies do seem to provoke some degree of public outcry. Moreover, as noted above, the *fear* of eugenics seems to motivate much of the public opposition to genetic manipulation that does exist. But how fair is the comparison between eugenics and contemporary forms of genetic intervention? It is an important question, and one that needs to be examined and reexamined as genetic technologies progress and develop.

Eugenics and "Genomics": A Comparison

Although there is no easy or direct parallel between the eugenics movement of the late nineteenth and early twentieth centuries, on the one hand, and today's efforts at human genetic manipulation, on the other, the two phenomena do not exist in isolation from one another. Indeed, in many respects human genetics itself emerged from the post–World War II, profoundly chastened field of eugenics. The two endeavors share many of the same general aims, attitudes, and social effects, though they also differ profoundly in terms of the means that they employ and the justifications that they offer. A comparison of the two reveals not that there is ample basis for our worst fears regarding the potential of a "slippery slope" in the direction of eugenic abuse, but rather that there are certain harmful tendencies to which we as a society seem prone, tendencies of which we should, minimally, be aware if we are to avoid repeating (albeit in different and perhaps more subtle ways) some of the more insidious errors of our past.

Similarities

Perhaps the most striking similarity between the early twentieth-century eugenics movement and the forms of genetic manipulation that are being developed at the start of the twenty-first century lies in a common aim: each represents an attempt to "better" the genetic heritage of humankind, or at least some subset of humankind. In other words, both aim to affect, in a "positive" direction, the kind of people who are born. Moreover, at least the *rhetoric* of both includes the goal of reducing the suffering of humankind and bettering the lives of society's future descendants. From Francis Galton's sense of duty toward the "future inhabitants of the earth," to Albert Wiggam's assertion that eugenics extends the Golden Rule "down the stream of protoplasm," the historical Anglo-American eugenics movement claims to have had human welfare at its heart. Even the leaders of the Nazi racial hygiene movement, which led to some of the worst horrors the world has ever witnessed, saw themselves as "guardian[s] of a millennial future" and their work as part of a "divine mission."[43]

I do not mean to suggest that the true aim of Nazi racial hygiene policy was the reduction of suffering; that would be a monstrous distortion. Rather, both Anglo-American eugenic thought and German racial hygiene ideology seem to have been infused with a utopian sense of purpose for ultimately bettering the human race, however horrific and cruel the means they sought to employ. Certainly, most contemporary geneticists do not appear to advance their cause with the same degree of spiritual fervor as did these earlier proponents. Nor are they as likely to stress the welfare of future generations as much as the alleviation of human suffering now. These are important distinctions. Still, contemporary proponents of genetic manipulation do share with their predecessors the urge to improve the human situation, present and future, using genetic means.[44]

In a related vein, one might say that both past eugenic efforts and current techniques of genetic manipulation implicitly include, on some level, a commitment to transform the population to reflect a specific set of social or even individual values. By this I do not mean that all proponents of genetic manipulation seek in the end to create a society of "perfect" human beings; rather, particular values (intelligence, beauty, diligence, health, etc.) are reflected in the visions put forth by various sorts of genetic "reformers." This is important to recognize, for the values themselves represent social or personal judgments of what constitutes a "good" life. Of course, these values are not identical across time. Nazi racial hygienists may have included a "Nordic" head shape in their list of positive values, whereas a modern-day proponent of gene manipulation might focus on the capacity for improved memory. Yet each choice represents particular values held by particular societies or individuals. As such, they are prone to the same discriminatory and self-advancing tendencies to which societies and individuals themselves are vulnerable. To wit, critic Gena Corea points out that in the case of early twentieth-century eugenics, " 'high quality' humans turned out to bear an astonishing resemblance to the eugenicists themselves."[45] Surely contemporary efforts at gene manipulation share this danger with their eugenic predecessors, even as they are employed to create a better world.

Aside from their aims, in what other respects do current endeavors in genetic manipulation resemble past eugenic efforts? Importantly, they both seem to be inclined to the danger of a deterministic worldview that holds heredity to be nearly all-powerful. This tendency is apparent enough in past eugenic efforts that attributed a huge variety of human behaviors, from poverty to trustworthiness, to simple heredity. Today, responsible scientists are the first to admit that heredity is complex and that the role of environment is at least as important as the role of genes in determining what a human person is like. Nevertheless, scientists have commonly constructed images for the genome — the "Book of Life," the "Holy Grail," a "Delphic oracle," or a "medical crystal ball" — that bolster a public perception of the gene as the all-determining force in the human character. Moreover, popular culture has transformed whatever grain of scientific truth there is in the determinative power of genes into an image of the gene as a complete source of identity — a convenient way to talk about personhood, guilt and responsibility, power and privilege, and intellectual or emotional status. Genes are popularly seen as responsible for everything from obesity and intelligence to criminality and shyness. In these respects, the gene of contemporary thought strongly resembles the "germplasm" of the early eugenics movements: "Indeed, the almost magical powers of the germplasm resonate in remarkable ways with those of the highly medicalized and specific gene of the 1990s."[46]

Such a deterministic view of genes undoubtedly contributes to a tendency to seek "better" babies via eugenic and/or genetic manipulation. Hence, early eugenic efforts share with contemporary genetics the danger of encouraging a view of children as little more than aggregates of inherited or intentionally designed characteristics to be shaped at will. If the gene, or the "germplasm," contains within it the blueprint for a human person, then manipulating genes (or germplasm) becomes an attractive means to control entire human persons, or even, in the minds of some, entire populations. The role of environment, and thus of social responsibility for environment, diminishes, and children become more squarely objects for conscious design.

A final way in which past eugenic movements and present-day efforts at genetic manipulation resemble each other is that both seem liable to exacerbate existent social injustices. Again, in the case of past efforts, the point is clear: beliefs about heredity were exploited to discriminate, often in extremely cruel ways, against poor people and other social "misfits." It is not unreasonable to fear that similar social injustice may be the logical result of contemporary efforts at genetic control. For instance, under current patterns of economic and healthcare distribution, the well-to-do are much more likely to avail themselves of genetic services, while the poor very likely will go untreated, potentially leading to exaggerated economic inequality. In this scenario it is easy to see how genetic disease could become localized in society's poorer communities. In a similar vein, some have described potential race-based discrimination in the realms of genetic screening, testing, and therapy.[47] Even though past discrimination in eugenics was largely driven by legislation and other forms of state control, it seems likely that relying on the free market for distribution of genetic services could also result in social injustice; the power of the market simply replaces the power of the state, favoring those with more money to spend.[48]

Dissimilarities

Despite these many, and sobering, similarities between past eugenic efforts and contemporary attempts at genetic manipulation, we must not be too quick to equate the two phenomena, for they do differ in crucial ways. To begin with, as noted above, eugenic policies of the past were enforced by the state, primarily by means of laws restricting the rights of individuals and groups. Since that time, a civil rights movement of enormous impact has intervened, and, in most Western societies at least, protections are now in place that simply did not exist in the early twentieth century. Among these is the public recognition of reproductive freedom, which now stands in the way of the worst abuses that eugenics proponents sought to implement. Moreover, the empowerment of many minority groups, including the disabled community, that began with the reforms of the 1960s and 1970s did much to work against the kind of state-sanctioned repression that characterized aspects of the earlier eugenics movement.

Because of these changes that have since taken place, any efforts at shaping our children that are likely to take place now will almost certainly be voluntary. Yet "voluntary" can be a slippery word; and, as many have pointed out, absolute freedom is a myth in any concrete social context, where social expectations and economic reality invariably moderate individual decisions. Hence, as Diane Paul holds, simply differentiating earlier forms of eugenics by their "coercive" character is, in the end, unhelpful, since coercion has different meanings in different social traditions; moreover, strongly held social values are always at least partially coercive on individuals.[49]

Still, there is a big difference between legislatively imposed, state-enforced eugenic action, on the one hand, and individual "eugenic" choices that are made with at least some degree of freedom, on the other. The technical forms of genetic manipulation that are a possibility (or a near possibility) today are a far cry from the widespread involuntary sterilization of the 1920s and 1930s. They are also a far cry from the high degree of state coordination required for the *Brave New World* scenarios envisioned by the most vociferous foes of gene manipulation. If we *are* on a slippery slope to eugenic abuse, it is difficult to imagine, at least in the United States, that it will take the road of openly coercive policies whereby the heavy-handed arm of the state represses the choices of individuals.

This point leads us to perhaps the most prominent difference between past eugenic movements and current attempts at genetic manipulation: the justifications that they offer are profoundly different. Past efforts at eugenic change relied heavily on *social* justifications: the betterment of society, the needs of the community, the well-being of future generations. This social emphasis is not absent in contemporary discussion, but it undoubtedly plays second fiddle to an emphasis on *individual* choice. Some of the most vociferous proponents of gene manipulation base their support primarily on the individual's right to choose or "design" the characteristics of their offspring, or simply to prevent suffering in their offspring when that seems likely. Interference with this individual choice is interpreted as intrusive and unwarranted. Indeed, many critics of past eugenic practices seem to believe that an ethic of radical individualism applied to reproductive decisions will protect current techniques of genetic manipulation from deteriorating into "eugenics" per se.[50]

It is exactly this individualist bent that may in fact make the new genetics more powerful and far-reaching. Whereas past eugenic ideals required heavy-handed social control over a number of generations for their implementation, newer genetic techniques could, in theory, allow change to occur rapidly and precisely, dramatically changing large numbers of individual children in any given generation.[51] Of course, other factors (e.g., cost) may well prevent this from occurring. Nevertheless, if genetic science were to advance to the level of precision hoped for in some circles, a very high degree of power to manipulate children's genomes — a power that could far exceed that of the less exact "science" of earlier forms of eugenics — could well be disseminated among millions of individuals, each exercising his or her individual reproductive choice.

Lessons from Our Past

What, if anything, is to be learned from these similarities and dissimilarities between past eugenic thought and present-day hopes for genetic manipulation? If the loudest critics of genetic technologies are correct, we are on a dangerous path — a slippery slope — to repeating eugenic abuse. Yet, as pointed out above, contemporary forms of shaping our offspring are in many ways quite different from eugenic efforts of the past, and U.S. society today has in place multiple safeguards against the kind of state-sanctioned repressive policies that marked early twentieth-century approaches. Moreover, very often the intention of those who wish to manipulate their children genetically is simply to prevent or reduce pain and suffering — quite a different story from the grand intentions of many eugenic reformers.

Perhaps the most important insight to be gained from the historical lesson is that we as a society seem to be prone to not tolerating imperfection in our progeny. The movements for eugenics in this century appear to have begun with a benevolent impulse to improve the lives of offspring, and to have twisted that impulse into a drive gradually to obliterate the less-than-perfect (however perceived) within the human species. Surely the inclination to improve a human being's life — to reduce her suffering, to encourage him to be all that he can be — is a praiseworthy one, but at some point advocates of eugenics seem to have crossed a line delineating appropriate limits in the quest for human betterment. If the history of eugenics teaches us nothing else, it should teach us to be attentive to our perfectionism and to be wary of the ways that it can lead us to do harm, obvious or subtle, to ourselves or others.

Another lesson to be learned from the history of eugenics is that we should remain vigilant about the effect of genetic technologies on social injustice. It seems clear that those who suffered most from the eugenic ideologies of the early twentieth century were poor people and other social "misfits" of the time; they became, as they so often do, scapegoats for society's woes. Today, as we increasingly see arguments in the public arena that mothers on welfare should be required, or very strongly encouraged, to make use of Norplant (or other, more permanent forms of birth control), we must question how far we as a society have really come since the days of forcible sterilization.[52] Genetic technologies could be a powerful way for society once again to live out its discriminatory patterns and to project certain of its values (health, strength, intelligence, beauty) at the expense of the poor and the socially weak.

Finally, an examination of the history of eugenics should lead us to challenge any deterministic worldview that holds that biology is destiny, and that altering our biology can in some way "fix" every human woe. Early eugenicists made the error of exaggerating the role of genetics in almost every conceivable human trait and behavior. As many today have pointed out, contemporary understanding runs a similar risk, tending to overstate the role of genetics and underemphasize that of environment in the development of disease and other aspects of human life. Overemphasizing the role of genetics in human character can lead to a passive attitude toward social injustice and a willingness to blame individuals rather than social structures for a multitude of social problems.[53] We have seen these patterns throughout the history of eugenics; we should be on guard against them as contemporary genetic techniques progress and develop.

In this regard, a final caveat: Certainly human beings *should not be reduced* to their genes; we are indeed far more than our genetic makeup. But human beings also *are not less* than their genetic makeup. Genes do play a crucial role in who we are, in the "givens" of our lives that we human beings must address. Hence, although we should not slip into biological determinism, attributing all human behavior to genes, we also should not underestimate the importance of genes to who we are and to our possibilities in life. Altering our children's genes will by no means solve every human woe, save the human race from deterioration, or ensure a bright future for our progeny. Perhaps it will not even make any sort of dent at all in our many intractable social problems. It could, however, profoundly alter the lives of many of our children and the "givens" that they must face as they negotiate their world. Hence, renouncing genetic determinism does not entail relinquishing moral responsibility for the powers of genetic manipulation that we now, or may soon, possess.

Pursuing Perfection: A Caution

This brief history of eugenic thought in Western society and the foregoing examination of perfectionist attitudes toward children in the United States today do not tell us how to respond to the burgeoning field of genetic manipulation of offspring. What they do tell us, however, is that we must not respond uncritically — that is, we must not respond as if there were no human precedent for the horrible atrocities that might result from the abuse of such technologies. The danger is real. The tendency to pursue perfection in the human race, even at enormous cost, is not merely a part of our past; it exists even today, albeit in an arguably more benign form, in our proclivity to desire "perfect" babies and children.

Yet these warnings should not cause us to entrench ourselves against all technological developments, as if ignoring or denouncing them will make them go away. The Pandora's box is open. Informed deliberation about policies concerning genetic manipulation, and about the possibility of "designer children," will depend, in part, upon wise and critical reflection about how these possibilities will affect us as a society. Such reflection in turn will suffer insofar as it fails to take account of the context of our perfectionist and consumerist present as well as our eugenic past. Hence, my hope is that the discussion to follow, in particular the normative recommendations I make, keeps this context very much in mind.

Notes

1. Leon R. Kass, *Toward a More Natural Science: Biology and Human Affairs* (New York: The Free Press, 1985), 62.
2. David Elkind, *The Hurried Child* (Menlo Park, Calif.: Addison-Wesley, 1981).
3. Nancy Ann Davis, "Reproductive Technologies and Our Attitudes Towards Children," *Logos* 9 (1988): 58.
4. It is not my purpose here to cast negative (or, for that matter, positive) judgment on the decision to abort a fetus known to be the carrier of the chromosomal error associated with Down syndrome. Indeed, a distinct lack of sufficient social services for persons with disabilities in U.S. society should at least cause us to pause before questioning a parent's decision to abort such a fetus. My point here is to highlight how the social proclivity to accept and even expect such an abortion, even without knowledge of the severity of the condition, seems to indicate, for whatever reason, a growing tendency to expect a child free from imperfection.
5. Ted Peters, *For the Love of Children: Genetic Technology and the Future of the Family* (Louisville: Westminster John Knox, 1996), 92.
6. Davis, "Reproductive Technologies," 61–62.
7. Ibid., 62.
8. LeRoy Walters and Julie Gage Palmer, *The Ethics of Human Gene Therapy* (New York: Oxford University Press, 1997), 131–32; Glenn McGee, *The Perfect Baby: A Pragmatic Approach to Genetics* (Lanham, Md.: Rowman & Littlefield, 1997), ix, 77.
9. Mary Winkler, cited in Erik Parens, "Is Better Always Good? The Enhancement Project," *The Hastings Center Report* 28, no. 1, special supplement (1998): S12.
10. Oliver O'Donovan, *Begotten or Made?* (Oxford: Clarendon, 1984), 73.
11. Gena Corea, *The Mother Machine: Reproductive Technologies from Artificial Insemination to Artificial Wombs* (New York: Harper & Row, 1985), 17.
12. Agneta Sutton, "The New Genetics: Facts, Fictions and Fears," *Linacre Quarterly* 62, no. 3 (1995): 85, 87.
13. Daniel J. Kevles, *In the Name of Eugenics: Genetics and the Uses of Human Heredity* (Cambridge, Mass.: Harvard University Press, 1995), 277.
14. Ibid., ix.

15. Francis Galton, *Inquiries into Human Faculty and Its Development* (New York: Macmillan, 1883), 24–25.

16. Francis Galton, *Hereditary Genius: An Inquiry into Its Laws and Consequences,* rev. ed. (New York: Appleton, 1891), 1.

17. Quoted in Edward J. Larson, *Sex, Race, and Science: Eugenics in the Deep South* (Baltimore: Johns Hopkins University Press, 1995), 19.

18. The fact that Galton's work is now considered to be only quasi-scientific should not obscure the fact that many of the most prominent supporters of the twentieth-century eugenics movement were leading biologists, and that eugenics itself is the forerunner of the present-day field of genetics.

19. Mark H. Haller, *Eugenics: Hereditarian Attitudes in American Thought* (New Brunswick, N.J.: Rutgers University Press, 1963), 3.

20. Kevles, *In the Name of Eugenics,* 49, 51. See also Donald K. Pickens, *Eugenics and the Progressives* (Nashville: Vanderbilt University Press, 1968), 57–59.

21. Kevles, *In the Name of Eugenics,* 59, 61.

22. Ibid., 97. On this tendency see Diane B. Paul, *Controlling Human Heredity: 1865 to the Present* (Atlantic Highlands, N.J.: Humanities Press, 1995), 97–98; Haller, *Eugenics,* 173–74.

23. Kevles, *In the Name of Eugenics,* 99; Haller, *Eugenics,* 142–43.

24. Philip R. Reilly, "Eugenic Sterilization in the United States," in *Contemporary Issues in Bioethics,* ed. Tom L. Beauchamp and LeRoy Walters (Belmont, Calif.: Wadsworth, 1994), 602. The state of Virginia had the second-highest number of sterilizations in the entire United States, trailing only California. In February 2001 the Virginia House of Delegates voted to express official regret for the state's role in the U.S. eugenics movement. See Craig Timberg, "Virginia House Regrets 'Eugenics,'" *San Francisco Chronicle,* February 4, 2001, A3, A8.

25. Steven Jay Gould, "Carrie Buck's Daughter," in Beauchamp and Walters, eds., *Contemporary Issues in Bioethics,* 610. Laughlin's views later were cited supportively by Fritz Lenz, leading racial hygiene theorist in Nazi Germany.

26. Marc Lappé, "Eugenics: Ethical Issues," in *Encyclopedia of Bioethics,* ed. Warren Thomas Reich, rev. ed. (New York: Simon & Schuster Macmillan, 1995), 772.

27. Kevles, *In the Name of Eugenics,* 118.

28. Robert Jay Lifton, "Sterilization and the Nazi Biomedical Vision," in Beauchamp and Walters, eds., *Contemporary Issues in Bioethics,* 621.

29. Ibid., 618, 620.

30. Ibid., 618; Stefan Kühl, *The Nazi Connection: Eugenics, American Racism, and German National Socialism* (New York and Oxford: Oxford University Press, 1994), 43. This point should not eclipse the existence of Christian opposition, vigorous at times, to much of Nazi policy (e.g., to euthanasia), particularly as time went on. Such opposition was especially true of the radical faction within that portion of the German Protestant Church often called the "Confessing Church," although it must also be remembered that this faction represented a distinct minority, even within Protestantism.

31. *Lebensborn* also supported special spa-like homes where racially desirable German women were urged to become pregnant by SS soldiers in order to bear "superior" babies. See Kevles, *In the Name of Eugenics,* 117; Robert Jay Lifton, *The Nazi Doctors: Medical Killing and the Psychology of Genocide* (New York: Basic Books, 1986), 43; Philip R. Reilly,

The Surgical Solution: A History of Involuntary Sterilization in the United States (Baltimore: Johns Hopkins University Press, 1991), 83.

32. Robert N. Proctor, *Racial Hygiene: Medicine Under the Nazis* (Cambridge, Mass.: Harvard University Press, 1988), 212, 207.

33. Ibid., 193.

34. Protestants, on the other hand, appear to have shown much less opposition to Anglo-American eugenic thought, at least in its heyday. Indeed, sympathizers of the social gospel movement also often sympathized with the eugenics movement and its ideals. See Haller, *Eugenics,* 83; Kevles, *In the Name of Eugenics,* 119.

35. Kevles, *In the Name of Eugenics,* 121, 199; Paul, *Controlling Human Heredity,* 119–20.

36. Kevles, *In the Name of Eugenics,*, 277.

37. Ibid., 270ff.

38. Daniel J. Kevles, "Eugenics: Historical Aspects," in Reich, ed., *Encyclopedia of Bioethics,* 769.

39. Lappé, "Eugenics," 774–75; see Troy Duster, *Backdoor to Eugenics* (New York: Routledge, 1990).

40. Kevles, "Eugenics: Historical Aspects," 767.

41. C. K. Chan, "Eugenics on the Rise: A Report from Singapore," in *Ethics, Reproduction and Genetic Control,* ed. Ruth F. Chadwick (New York: Routledge, 1992), 165.

42. Kevles, "Eugenics: Historical Aspects," 767–68; Robert N. Proctor, "Genomics and Eugenics: How Fair Is the Comparison?" in *Gene Mapping: Using Law and Ethics as Guides,* ed. George J. Annas and Sherman Elias (New York: Oxford University Press, 1992), 93 n. 108.

43. Lifton, "Sterilization," 614, 620.

44. Gene therapy pioneer W. French Anderson has been a most articulate spokesperson for the urgency of the goal of reduced suffering. In his words, "The 'rush' [for gene therapy trials] arises from our human compassion for our fellow man who needs help now. . . . The sooner we begin, the sooner patients will be helped." Quoted in Leon Jaroff, "Battler for Gene Therapy," *Time,* January 17, 1994, 57.

45. Corea, *Mother Machine,* 20.

46. Dorothy Nelkin and M. Susan Lindee, *The DNA Mystique: The Gene as Cultural Icon* (New York: W. H. Freeman, 1995), 5–7, 16, 36.

47. See, for example, Duster, *Backdoor to Eugenics;* Patricia A. King, "The Past as Prologue: Race, Class, and Gene Discrimination," in Annas and Elias, eds., *Gene Mapping,* 94–111.

48. Diane B. Paul, "Eugenic Anxieties, Social Realities, and Political Choices," in *Are Genes Us? The Social Consequences of the New Genetics,* ed. Carl F. Cranor (New Brunswick, N.J.: Rutgers University Press, 1994), 152.

49. Ibid., 146; Philip Kitcher, *The Lives to Come: The Genetic Revolution and Human Possibilities* (New York: Simon & Schuster, 1996), 199.

50. Paul, "Eugenic Anxieties," 154.

51. Robert L. Sinsheimer, "The Prospect of Designed Genetic Change," in Chadwick, ed., *Ethics, Reproduction and Genetic Control,* 144.

52. "Tennessee Eyes Reward for Birth Control," *San Francisco Chronicle,* April 17, 1992, A9; Karen Southwick, "Use Norplant, Don't Go to Jail," *San Francisco Chronicle,* August 2, 1992, Z1/13; Dorothy Roberts, "Norplant's Threat to Civil Liberties and Racial Justice," *New Jersey Law Journal* 134, no. 13 (1993): 20.

53. Nelkin and Lindee, *The DNA Mystique,* 101. The search for the "crime gene," which has surfaced and resurfaced over the years, is one example of the many misguided attempts to connect human behavior too closely with genetic predisposition. See Suzuki and Knudtson, *Genethics,* chapter 6; Kevles, *In the Name of Eugenics,* 46–47, 71. Recent findings that the aggregate number of human genes may be much lower than previously thought should cause us to reject genetic determinism even more vigorously.

Chapter Three

Choosing Children

Feminism and the Place of Procreative Liberty

> *There is no doubt that individualism, like salt, is a very good and necessary thing, and that the eighteenth-century thinkers did quite right to shout for it. They provided a real Enlightenment. But how about a diet of salt alone? . . . Unmitigated individualism is a death-wish.*
>
> — Mary Midgley and Judith Hughes[1]

In the face of today's massive changes in human influence over reproduction, one norm stands out, in scholarly and popular media, as a means of sorting through the ensuing muddle of moral quandaries: the norm of procreative liberty. Procreative liberty typically is held up by liberal theorists as the central framework from which to make ethical determinations about new reproductive and genetic technologies. This should come as no surprise, for liberal[2] thinkers often tend to privilege individual freedom to a high degree, viewing it as the sine qua non of what it means to be human. Liberal thought in regard to genetic manipulation is no exception, maintaining that any restraint upon individual procreative liberty conveys a disrespect for individuals themselves.

It is not, however, liberal theorists alone who traditionally have elevated the norm of procreative liberty. It has also been something of a rallying cry in twentieth-century feminism. Described at various points as "reproductive freedom," "procreative choice," or simply "our right to choose," the norm generally is invoked to defend women's right to control their own bodies and procreative capacities, including their access to safe and legal abortion services. Not all feminists, of course, embrace the concept of procreative liberty with equal fervor, but undeniably it has gained a privileged position in feminist discourse, and typically it is understood as foundational to, if not a guarantor of, women's well-being in society.

Given the strength of such claims about procreative liberty, it is imperative that we evaluate its role in regard to the possibility of "designing" our children. Should individuals be granted unlimited access to these technologies, such that the norm of procreative liberty carries the day? In the present chapter I first will examine "strong" claims of procreative liberty — claims, both liberal and feminist, that make a privileged place for personal freedom in reproductive choices. Although these two approaches bear some similarities to one another, a comparison of them reveals that feminism, even in its less radical forms, adds distinctive emphases to the discussion that will prove crucial to further moral evaluation. In other words, feminism ideally carries us beyond a single-minded emphasis on procreative liberty to a more comprehensive vision, one that privileges not just procreative liberty, but also a more substantive and contextual understanding of human well-being. This vision itself begins to illuminate the direction in which we must move as we make decisions, individually and socially, about "designing" our children.

Liberal Approaches to "Designing" Children

Procreative Liberty and "Children of Choice"

In its clearest and most straightforward form, a strongly "liberal" approach to procreative liberty may be summarized as "the freedom to decide whether or not to have offspring and to control the use of one's reproductive capacity."[3] It is a freedom held by individuals and that extends to matters of conception, gestation and labor, and childrearing. Indeed, its most avid supporters rely on procreative liberty to justify a variety of procedures and practices ranging from therapeutic interventions and sex selection to cloning, and even at times to the intentional diminishment of offspring — in other words, "designing" children to possess qualities ordinarily considered to be undesirable or even harmful.

Among the most ardent supporters of this strong conception of procreative liberty is legal theorist John Robertson. Robertson understands procreative liberty to be ultimately rooted in its close connection to an individual's sense of meaning and identity, and in the profound importance that reproductive decisions carry for individuals. According to Robertson, part of living a fulfilled life, for many individuals, includes the ability to have "normal, healthy offspring" whom one intends to rear. "Reproduction," he writes, "occupies a central position in the lives of many people who consider reproduction meaningful only if the child they produce has certain characteristics such as good health." Hence, procreative liberty rightly safeguards actions designed to enable couples to have such offspring in their pursuit of personal fulfillment; as such, it must be protected. Indeed, in this regard, genetic technologies only enhance the freedom that individuals already possess to pursue "children of choice"; for in fact "parents often select mates in part with an eye to the vigor or beauty of their expected offspring and . . . go to extraordinary lengths through education and rearing to mold children to their image of perfection."[4]

Predictably, such arguments lead to a wide acceptance of the freedom to shape our offspring, and thereby to secure "children of choice," even by genetic means. In other words, the right to have offspring generally also entitles one to have offspring with particular characteristics. For Robertson, this is especially true if the decision to have children in the first place *depends* on the ability to choose the characteristics of those children. If this is the case, then the protection of procreative liberty itself demands that we also protect parental *choice* of offspring characteristics. In this way, Robertson justifies nearly every form of genetic manipulation imaginable — therapeutic manipulation, sex selection, nontherapeutic enhancement, most forms of cloning, and intentional diminishment (e.g., the "designing" of deaf children or children of extremely short stature).[5] On the one hand, procreative liberty protects parental choice, which is closely bound up with the decision to procreate in the first place; on the other hand, procreative liberty allows us to "better equip the child for life's perilous journey, and thus to assure that it will be happy and successful."[6]

One would expect that procreative liberty, so described, would exist as one value among many and so would have its limits in a democratic society. And yet, though Robertson does acknowledge that such limits may exist, in reality they are, for him, very few. A given practice must demonstrably lead to substantial and unavoidable harm to, or burden on, concrete individuals in order for procreative liberty to be justifiably overridden.[7] In other words, it is not enough for a practice to carry with it merely "symbolic" dangers to society or to groups within society — for instance the "symbolic" harm of endangering a particular image of the family (e.g., a two-parent family), or that of objectifying women or children as a group. In general, Robertson holds that, in a public and pluralistic setting, fundamental individual rights must supersede the broader conceptions of the good embodied in such concerns. Hence, the harm that ordinarily could justify the curtailment of individual procreative liberty is direct, tangible harm to others, not harm to the social value structure or offenses to personal conceptions of morality. Indeed, even the need for social justice "is not a compelling reason for limiting the procreative choice of those who can pay."[8]

Procreative Liberty in Feminist Accounts

It is here where liberals such as Robertson differ from liberals of a more feminist stripe. Feminists, even liberal feminists, tend to express greater concern about general social values as well as about specific harm to women threatened by genetic technologies. Although it is hard to nail down exactly what counts as "feminist" in contemporary ethical discourse, a common thread undoubtedly remains in the shared belief that women have been and are an oppressed group in most societies on account of their gender. Moreover, this oppression is not merely manifested in concrete harm to individual women; rather, it is embodied in social institutions and practices on a broader scale. Indeed, for those people ordinarily classified as liberal feminists, the assurance of procreative liberty often is seen as a modern milestone in working toward the goal of reducing this oppression.

A strongly feminist, and yet arguably still liberal, view of procreative liberty would privilege the right of individual women (and men) to make their own decisions about the "highly personal" matter of reproduction — a right that is particularly fragile and under attack in today's world. Women's control over their own reproduction is indeed hard-fought, and the historical denial of such control — for example, in the form of involuntary sterilizations and unnecessary hysterectomies or Cesarean sections, or of denied access to safe contraception and reproductive services — is a context that we must not too soon or too easily forget. In light of this dangerous history, reproductive freedom carries with it a particular significance for women, and feminists rightly worry that any denial of that freedom might represent the erosion of women's freedom more generally as well as a challenge to their concrete well-being.

One feminist theorist who argues along these lines is Mary Anne Warren. Warren has written primarily on the topic of sex selection, though it is possible to speculate how her arguments might be extended to other forms of shaping our offspring.[9] She acknowledges the power of many different objections to sex selection, including many of the objections raised in the first chapter of this book; yet none of the feared negative consequences of sex selection are likely enough to occur, in her view, to merit a breach of individual reproductive choice. In other words, the moral presumption in favor of freedom, she argues, is not easily outweighed, even by potentially harmful effects. Moreover, according to Warren, even the objection that sex selection objectifies children is misguided, for in practicing of sex selection, one does not necessarily equate the child's worth with his or her gender. Rather, one may wish to choose a child's sex for a variety of nonsexist reasons — for instance, the desire of parents to have both girls and boys. Hence, in Warren's view, such concerns do not represent significant challenges to honoring reproductive freedom. Even with other sorts of genetic manipulation, whether therapeutic or enhancement interventions, Warren urges us not to reject them out of hand, but rather to evaluate each on a case-by-case basis according to individual and social consequences. Only those with predictable, and predictably serious, consequences merit an overriding of procreative liberty, which she considers to be fundamental to human, and especially to women's, well-being.

These strong views of procreative liberty, feminist and nonfeminist alike, share much in common. Most outstanding is the individualism that marks the work of each; for both, the individual (or the individual couple) is the primary bearer of reproductive claims, claims that cannot easily be overridden by broader social needs or the quality of our common life. Moreover, each interprets the more general claim of respect for persons as dictating such a protection of procreative liberty under a rubric of basic individual rights.

These approaches also share a fairly similar view of the limits that they would impose on procreative liberty. Importantly, they emphasize that procreative liberty is most clearly limited by a substantial, concrete harm or burden to other individuals that can be predicted with a reasonable degree of certainty. Along similar lines, they agree that many of the fears commonly raised about genetic manipulation or sex selection are unlikely or, at a minimum, uncertain actually to occur. For both, the hypothetical negative consequences of a practice in the future must not be allowed to outweigh a strong right to procreative liberty in the present. In like manner, strongly liberal views such as these are apt to reject arguments that hold that genetic manipulation is somehow "unnatural" or a means of "playing God." Rather, they hold that part of human nature is in fact to exert control over nature itself. Further, they

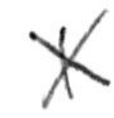

agree that the danger of objectifying a child is insufficient to override a commitment to procreative liberty.

Despite these points of agreement, a highly significant difference must be recognized: feminist liberals, more than the others, pay earnest and sustained attention to the consequences for women of reproductive practices and policies. It is true that they may be finally willing to override potential (if uncertain) social changes that could negatively affect women — for instance, changes in women's social circumstances as a class that could result from sex selection. Nevertheless, they are bound to take such concerns seriously and to pay significant attention to the historical and social context that may affect the likelihood of them coming to fruition.

A critical aspect of what feminism adds to a liberal discussion of procreative liberty, then, is enhanced consideration of women's well-being. Indeed, this sort of mindfulness is a crucial part of an analysis of genetic manipulation, for there can be little doubt that genetic technologies, like reproductive technologies generally, will have a disproportionately strong impact on the lives of women. Yet the emphasis on the need to protect women's reproductive choice, on the one hand, and consideration of the concrete consequences of these technologies for women, on the other, point toward a deep tension in liberal feminism between the "good" of reproductive liberty and the substantive well-being of persons, including women. Liberal feminists may, in fact, resolve this tension too readily by discounting concerns about potential harm to women. Indeed, the tension itself calls for a deeper analysis of the relationship between personal autonomy and concrete human well-being; clearly, the two do not always coincide.

Beyond Pure Procreative Liberty: Feminist Challenges to Liberal Accounts

Procreative liberty surely plays an important, even critical, role in evaluating the genetic manipulation of offspring characteristics. Moreover, feminists generally are loathe to cast aside the value of procreative liberty, for most agree that it has proved crucial in women's ongoing struggle to overcome their oppression. Yet strongly liberal accounts like those described above ultimately leave one unsatisfied, for such accounts contradict, to a greater or lesser degree, the intuition that there are stricter limits to be placed on how we should manipulate human reproduction. The central problem with these liberal accounts lies finally in the nearly absolute authority that they grant to individual autonomy at the expense of other significant dimensions of human life.

Feminist thought has been at the forefront of this recognition. Of course, a diversity of feminist theory exists; today one rightly must speak of "feminisms," in the plural. Nevertheless, certain ethical values and concerns seem to reappear with some degree of consistency across many different types of contemporary feminist thinking—a "short list" does include autonomy, but also, importantly, such values as relationality (including equality and mutuality) and embodiment. Minimally we can say that a significant strand of feminist thought promotes some version of these values as important components of human well-being.

Again, not all feminists embrace these values or even speak about them directly, and certainly any given feminist theorist will differentially emphasize one or another of them in an effort to construct an adequate feminist ethic. Yet they do provide a basis of sorts for a feminist approach to genetic manipulation. Moreover, it is especially noteworthy that autonomy does not stand alone in feminist thought as the sole, or even the most important, component of human well-being. Autonomy, to be sure, crucially underlies the respect due human persons generally and women in particular, and as such it is a critical component of well-being. Yet an overemphasis on autonomy can lead to an exaggerated individualism, one that distorts our concrete, embodied existence, whereby we are profoundly embedded in familial and social relationships. These relationships shape and define the choices that we make, and indeed our very being. To ignore or downplay them, as strong liberals are prone to do, is to misconstrue and falsify the human experience.

Human well-being and women's well-being depend on more than promoting autonomy. In the words of Christian theologian Elizabeth A. Johnson, feminist theology's rejection of women's oppression is grounded in a "deep and lasting *yes* to women's flourishing"—that is, to women's well-being as a whole, to their *full humanity*.[10] An adequate understanding of women's well-being—indeed, of human well-being—moves far beyond unrestricted individual choice; it embraces and attends to both our autonomy and our relationality, including our status as embodied persons and our insertion into familial, social, and cultural contexts.

Hence, when we evaluate different approaches to genetic manipulation, we must indeed examine whether or not they protect individual autonomy, and, in particular, reproductive autonomy for women. This aspect of women's well-being must not be overlooked. Crucially, however, we must also examine whether the manipulations themselves promote and enhance human well-being more fully considered. From a feminist standpoint, of course, this includes especially the well-being of women.[11] It also includes the well-being of children, for three reasons: first, children are perhaps the most directly affected by the technologies in question; second, in most societies, including our own, women are related to children in a most intimate way, both physically and socially; and third, feminism as a whole maintains a special commitment to the well-being of those with severely limited social power — arguably, in this case, children. Finally, taking account of human well-being requires an examination of the impact of genetic manipulation on socioeconomic relations, whether or not it is likely to exacerbate harmful social patterns. All of these considerations merit further discussion, with an eye toward upholding the feminist values outlined above.

Reproductive Autonomy and Women's Well-Being

Most feminists agree that reproductive autonomy is an important component of women's well-being, and in addition that women have achieved some significant and hard-won gains in reproductive autonomy over the past half-century. Beverly Wildung Harrison speaks for many when she argues that the controversy over abortion has been but a most visible aspect of the larger struggle of women for full "procreative choice" — a struggle whose goals include access to safer contraception, greater economic and social security, stronger support for childrearing, lessening of racial brutality, and a reduction of violence against women. Although full procreative choice is still no more than a distant hope for most women, safe and legal abortion, in Harrison's view, provides at least the negative means of assuring the elements of such choice.[12]

It must be remembered that it was not always so for women. Relatively (though still not perfectly) safe and reliable forms of contraception are a fairly recent development, and limited access to abortion itself has been legal in the United States only since 1973. Yet contraception and abortion form only part of the picture; patriarchy's ignominious history includes a long chronicle of male control over women's reproductive capacities. Barbara Ehrenreich and Deirdre English have extensively described the gradual removal of the birth process from the hands of women, over the last 150 years, by a male-dominated medical profession.[13] Even today, it is women who, by and large, must choose to cope with their fertility, must take major responsibility for contraception, and must bear the brunt of childrearing in a society where their social power is limited and their life choices often are heavily constrained. The limited amount of procreative liberty that women enjoy today must be seen in the context of a long and ongoing struggle to claim control over their own reproductive lives *and* a wider context of deep-seated and long-standing patterns of male supremacy over women.

In Harrison's view, the capacity to shape their procreative power is a social good foundational to women's well-being; as such, it is part of the basic conditions necessary for a good society. To ensure procreative choice is simultaneously to recognize women as full moral agents, with serious moral claims to well-being, respect, self-direction, and noncoercion in childbearing. Furthermore, it is to recognize and acknowledge the actual social vulnerability of women, rooted in a concrete history of subjugation, particularly in relation to childbearing.[14] In this context, procreative choice must indeed be viewed as a critically important aspect of women's well-being, necessary to women's flourishing.

Yet it is worth highlighting that feminists (such as Harrison) who identify less as liberals and more as "radical" or "socialist" feminists,[15] while maintaining some form of procreative liberty as a positive good for women, also tend to expand the understanding of procreative freedom beyond negative liberty to include a more substantive vision of women's reproductive well-being. Additionally, some have pointed out that reproductive freedom exists in a social context that itself structures and defines women's choices. For instance, sociologist Barbara Katz Rothman defends the value of individual choice, but she simultaneously argues that purely free, unstructured choice is an illusion, since social forces in fact shape the alternatives available to individuals and influence their perceived needs. In this way, "as 'choices' become available, they all too rapidly become compulsions to 'choose' the socially endorsed alternative."[16]

Furthermore, certain freely made choices may over time erode other alternatives that previously had been available. For example, as Rothman points out, everyday travel by means of horse and carriage is functionally a nonoption in Western society today, where the automobile enjoys pervasive acceptance and use. Along similar lines, "in gaining the choice to control the quality of our children, we may rapidly lose the choice not to control the quality, the choice of simply accepting them as they are."[17] That is, the choice to control the "quality" of children (whether by means of amniocentesis and selective abortion, or, in the future, by means of genetic manipulation), as it becomes increasingly socially acceptable, may ultimately deprive us of the choice to forgo such measures entirely — that is, the choice to accept children unconditionally. In this light, "choice" should be viewed with a critical eye and a willingness to recognize that our liberty is always conditioned, since we simply cannot extricate ourselves from the very limiting concrete context in which we live as real, embodied persons. Our "right" to make choices does not exist in a vacuum, and our autonomy ultimately must be situated into, and indeed must serve, the larger category of human well-being. This is true for women as it is true for all human persons.

Embodied Relationality and the Well-Being of Women and Children

"Embodiment" and "relationality," two terms that appear throughout feminist theory, defy easy definition. *Embodiment* is, in part, a rejection of the traditional mind/body dualism that has so heavily characterized Western thought, especially since Descartes. To be embodied is to be a "whole" human being, not simply a rational mind housed in a body. Because women historically have been more associated with the body and men with the mind, and because this association has proved harmful and oppressive for women, feminist interpretation of embodiment began with the recognition and assertion that women are not to be any more associated with the body (or physical matter, or sexuality, or emotions) than men are, and that women, like men, can transcend the body through rational choice. Ethicist Margaret Farley points out that this move paradoxically freed women to take their bodies more seriously and eventually led to a feminist movement to reclaim the body as integral to selfhood. Concretely, this entails both an effort to take women's bodies seriously and to refuse to yield control of them to men.[18]

Whatever else it may mean, honoring embodiment implies the recognition that we are not simply rational minds inhabiting or owning bodies that are of secondary importance; rather, we are nothing if we are not body-selves and body-subjects. Focusing on rational choice as the primary moral arena and indeed as a way to "transcend" the limitations of the body (as might be proposed with technologies that allow us to shape and mold our children) runs the risk of denying our human embodiment to a dangerous degree. Indeed, this is precisely the tendency of many liberal feminists who weight human rationality and the value of choice so heavily that they tend to ignore or downplay the claims and needs of human bodies. As others have pointed out, liberal feminism does little to challenge the mind/body dualism embedded in liberal philosophy, and thus has no place for the inherent physicality of the processes of birth, lactation, and the "menial" work of body maintenance.[19] Likewise, liberal approaches to genetic manipulation are too quick to embrace choice, even when it may threaten women's (and children's) concrete, *embodied* well-being.

A more adequate approach to human embodiment takes the bodies of all persons, including most especially women and children, with great seriousness. Not only must we refrain from intervening in bodily processes without adequate justification, but also we must beware of damaging bodies in the course of whatever interventions we do undertake. Moreover, we must recognize that changes we might make to bodies (e.g., genetic manipulation of children's bodies) can have profound effects on the human persons involved because, again, bodies are not peripheral to human identity. Finally, and particularly germane to the issue of genetic manipulation, we do well to remember the diversity of human bodies in the world and the cultural constructedness of the idea of the "perfect" body.

Relationality is a value closely aligned with embodiment, for bodies do not exist in social isolation, but rather incarnate our human interdependence. Pregnancy is, of course, the quintessential example of human relationality; indeed, "we have in every pregnant woman the living proof that individuals do not enter the world as autonomous, atomistic, isolated beings, but begin socially, begin connected."[20] Part of being embodied means that we are not free-floating choice-makers, but rather bodies who live under concrete circumstances and in intimate relations with others — that is, in interpersonal, familial, and sociocultural contexts. Our relationality is an integral part of who we are and in large part, though not exclusively, even *defines* who we are: our possibilities, desires, and hopes for ourselves as well as our limitations and struggles.

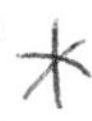

It is readily apparent that our relationality crucially constitutes (or, alternatively, contradicts) our well-being; as human persons we cannot be well at all if we are not well in our relations. Farley has highlighted the fact that our relationality underlies our ability to know and be known, to love and be loved, thus allowing us both self-transcendence and self-possession.[21] So understood, relationality, like autonomy, serves our human well-being. To honor human relationality means, among other things, to take our social embeddedness seriously, and to protect and attend to the many relationships that constitute any one person's social context. In the case of genetic manipulation it means to consider carefully the consequences of any proposed genetic technology on our interpersonal, familial, and social relations, and to uphold, insofar as possible, the values of equality and mutuality, which in turn promote human well-being.

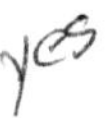

The terms "equality" and "mutuality," like "embodiment" and "relationality," require further delineation. *Equality* here refers primarily to the contemporary insight that women are not properly the moral or social inferiors of men, but rather, like men, deserve to be respected as ends in themselves and as bearers of full and equivalent human dignity. Obviously this principle is closely connected to that of autonomy, and indeed in its more liberal formulations simply extends individual autonomy and the capacity for free choice (classically liberal features of personhood) to women. Yet I include it here under the category of relationality because equality, in the sense of equal respect for women as persons, has obvious and dramatic relational implications, implications that challenge a socioeconomic system that still largely, even if sometimes implicitly, privileges men over women. To honor and uphold women's equality is to pose a marked challenge to many, if not most, social relationships as they exist in our world today. Indeed, feminism insists that women's well-being ultimately depends in part on just such a challenge.

The principle of equality is further fleshed out in a feminist proposal for equitable sharing. By way of this insight, some versions of feminist thought extend equality beyond the liberal, formal requirement of respect for persons to the larger assertion that all persons possess a legitimate claim to an equitable share in the goods and services necessary to human life and basic happiness. Hence, this represents not just a claim of equality of respect or even equality of opportunity, but rather a claim on all to recognize and participate in human solidarity. Although the precise structure of equitable sharing and the analysis of how it might best be achieved differ among feminists, there is nevertheless reasonably consistent opposition among feminists to stark socioeconomic inequalities wherein classes of people lack basic goods necessary to human well-being. Such vast inequalities are, according to feminist thought, a violation of human flourishing.

On a more interpersonal level, the feminist principle of *mutuality* may be said to be among the most consistently promoted components of relational well-being. Mutuality, as described well by feminist theologian

Elizabeth Johnson, "signifies a relation marked by equivalence between persons, a concomitant valuing of each other, a common regard marked by trust, respect, and affection in contrast to competition, domination, or assertions of superiority."[22] In other words, mutuality involves not a unidirectional submission of one to another, but rather a reciprocal relation wherein both parties engage in an affirmation of the other and a shared accountability to the demands of the relationship.[23] So understood, mutuality is marked by collaboration rather than competition, cooperative power ("power with") rather than possessive or dominative power ("power over"), and equality rather than hierarchy. In fact, it might be asserted that full mutuality is possible *only* in relations marked by equality. In mutual love, which is seen by many feminist theological ethicists as the deepest and most radical form of love, each party engages in an active affirmation of the beauty and goodness of the other, simultaneously receiving and giving within the love relationship.[24]

Mutuality is a key norm of relationships in feminist thought because it is in mutual relationships that human beings flourish. That is, to be involved in a relationship characterized by domination and submission or by a possessive attitude of one toward another is, according to feminist thought, unconducive to human well-being, including the well-being of both dominated and dominator. Promoting human well-being vis-à-vis genetic manipulation involves guarding against technologies that tend to encourage such destructive, nonmutual patterns of relationship.

In sum, upholding the norms of embodiment and relationality is a crucial part of what it means to honor women's and children's well-being. Yet it would be mistaken to think that these norms may be further elaborated or applied in the abstract; we must now turn more directly to the concrete circumstances of genetic manipulation and examine how women's and children's well-being—that is, their embodied, relational well-being—is best fostered.

The Well-Being of Women

In an essay entitled "Patriarchal Designs," feminist philosopher Shelley Minden reminds us that genetic technologies will have a special and dramatic impact on women: "One thing that is certain is the first people to be affected will surely be *women*, whose eggs, wombs, and lives will form the raw material for [the genetic engineering of the human embryo]."[25] Not only will women's bodies be directly affected by technologies of genetic manipulation, but because it is ordinarily women who assume primary responsibility for children in this society, it is these same women who most likely will bear any burdensome outcomes that result from the genetic manipulation of children. That is, in a society with few social supports for childrearing, it is primarily women whose lives will be changed.

Liberal thinkers, as noted above, are notorious for ignoring or subordinating considerations of substantive well-being, including, in this case, the concrete dangers posed to women as a result of various sorts of genetic manipulation. Among the most disturbing of these potential dangers is that technologies of genetic manipulation will extend the (historically sometimes harmful) power of medicine and technology even more deeply into women's lives. Feminists fear that this will further remove from women the locus of control over their bodies and health. Theorist Robyn Rowland voices this concern: "Increased technological intervention into the processes by which women conceive is increasing the male-dominated medical profession's control of procreation and will lead inevitably to greater social control of women by men."[26] To recognize this danger is simultaneously to recognize that women's concrete history and context is the history and context of patriarchy; patriarchy forms women's reality. Even as historical advancements in medicine, particularly reproductive medicine, have sometimes benefited women, they also have meant the greater insertion of the medical establishment, largely comprised of men, into the details of women's lives, and this medicalization generally has translated into a history of great pain for women, particularly in the areas of pregnancy and childbirth. A long list of medical abuses against women — from medically unnecessary hysterectomies and cesarean sections to the disastrous prescription of diethylstilbestrol (DES) to hundreds of thousands of women, resulting in infertility and even cancer in their daughters — confirms the fear: women must not be

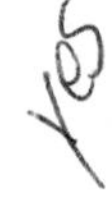

overly sanguine about the contributions of medicine to their overall well-being. A commitment to honoring embodiment demands that genetic technologies be developed and implemented using only the greatest of care vis-à-vis women's (and children's) bodies, particularly in light of medicine's disgraceful history with respect to women's well-being.

It is not only women's bodily well-being, of course, that is threatened by genetic technologies; women's psychological/emotional well-being also faces potential challenges. If contemporary infertility treatment is any indication of what the implementation of genetic technologies will be like for women, the future does not look bright. Lisa Sowle Cahill describes the objectification and humiliation that are commonly part of women's infertility treatment:

> Even if sexual banter and phallic references among physicians are more rare than some critics report, teams which prod and inspect a prone woman, feet in stirrups, genitals exposed, all the while discussing ways in which she can be made pregnant, reduce her to a state of sexual humiliation.[27]

Of course, presently it is unclear exactly *how* technologies of genetic manipulation would be implemented; whether or not procedures would take place on pregnant women's bodies remains to be seen. Yet, at a minimum, the strong possibility exists that the bodies of pregnant women will be further objectified as they submit to procedures designed to "improve" the quality of their offspring. According to an adequate understanding of human embodiment, such bodily objectification is far from insignificant, but rather can profoundly affect women's overall (including psychological/emotional) well-being.

Related to such fears is the feminist concern that technologies of genetic manipulation will conduce to the further commodification of reproduction, and simultaneously to potentially degrading views of women in general, as well as to disembodying, dehumanizing reproductive experiences. Some have described a trend whereby prenatal testing encourages us to think of pregnancy differently: babies and children are increasingly viewed as products, and mothers as producers; pregnant women are akin to unskilled workers on a reproductive assembly line.[28] It goes without saying that the effort to predetermine children's characteristics will only exacerbate such a trend. The prospect of "designing" children carries with it the danger that women will increasingly come to be viewed as breeders, identified largely with their reproductive capacities. Moreover, it seems likely that the implementation of genetic manipulation will further fragment the experiences of conception, gestation, and birth, as women (very likely undergoing in vitro fertilization) are subtly encouraged to consider the process as a series of steps toward producing a particular *kind* of child. At a minimum, a feminist ethic must challenge such a fragmentation of the reproductive experience as subtly disembodying, and thus as contrary to women's flourishing.

These harms to women may not be concrete, tangible, or easily identifiable in any given case, but nevertheless they pose a real danger. Any inclination to dismiss harms such as these as merely "symbolic" is highly disturbing when considered from a feminist standpoint. Indeed, one may validly call into question why "symbolic" harm should be thought of as insignificant, especially in a society where images seem to have the power to shape human consciousness generally. In other words, "attention to women's experience has taught feminists that there are no 'merely symbolic' harms; we interpret and shape experience through our symbols and therefore how we think about persons, events, and biological processes has a great deal to do with how we behave toward them.[29] Accordingly, an approach to genetic manipulation that seeks to foster women's well-being *on all levels* will take seriously indeed the changes wrought by genetic technologies on our social understanding of reproduction, including the degree to which it is appropriately commodified, and on women's role in the reproductive process.

There is yet another way in which access to technologies that allow parents to genetically "design" their children might disproportionately affect women. As noted above, in contemporary society it is primarily women who take care of, and take primary responsibility for, children. It may be that the option to choose offspring characteristics may well increase the burden of responsibility on individual parents, and in particular on mothers, to a nearly intolerable level. In other words, not only will parents, especially mothers, be responsible for children's upbringing, but also they will begin to be viewed (and to view themselves) as ultimately responsible for many different aspects of children's genetic health (or illness), intelligence level, and personality characteristics, insofar as these are understood to be influenced by genes. High expectations on the part of spouses or even society in general undoubtedly will add to whatever personal pressure potential mothers are likely to place upon themselves. Moreover, insofar as individual mothers (and fathers) are seen as responsible for genetic "defects" in their children, society apparently is released from any collective responsibility for the care and accommodation of those who are born less than "perfect" — for example, children with cystic fibrosis or of a lesser intelligence level. In some cases, of course, genetic manipulation could free mothers from heavy burdens that otherwise must be born largely alone — for instance, the emotional and financial burden of caring for a child with serious genetic illness. Yet this gain may come at the cost of individualizing responsibility for problems, placing a weighty responsibility indeed on the shoulders of all parents with less-than-perfect children.

Sex Preselection and Women's Flourishing: Some Special Considerations

The foregoing considerations may apply to many different forms of genetic manipulation, and certainly to the three case studies addressed in this book. Genetic manipulation for the prevention of cystic fibrosis, for the enhancement of memory, and for sex preselection all run the risk of being implemented in a way that threatens the bodily and psychological/emotional well-being of women; these technologies also may contribute to the overall commodification of reproduction and to dehumanizing views and treatment of women. Finally, each would likely increase the burden of responsibility experienced by individual parents, especially mothers, for the "quality" of their children.

Yet there are additional considerations of women's well-being that arise specifically in the case of sex preselection. To begin with, as noted above, many feminists fear potential threats to women's social status resulting from the widespread practice of sex preselection. In many parts of the world it appears highly likely that sex preselection technologies will raise the male-female sex ratio, in some cases dramatically. This could further diminish the status of women, confining them more easily to subordinate and traditionally "feminine" roles. Indeed, even Warren acknowledges that there is some empirical evidence that high sex-ratio societies tend to hinder women's well-being because they tend to be severely patriarchal, confining women to domestic roles and limiting their interactions with men. After describing this argument in some detail, Warren concludes that the evidence does not justify any strong predictions; she believes that too much depends on the particular details of individual societies, especially the degree of structural power that men hold to begin with.[30] Others disagree, however, highlighting in particular the likelihood that "scarce" women will be valued for sexual and breeding purposes rather than for their intrinsic worth as persons. In the words of one theorist, "Women are the most exploited, manipulated, oppressed and brutalized group in the world, yet we have the numbers. What would our status be as a vastly outnumbered group? And how many women would be prepared to accept a world where their value as breeders or sexual objects only would be recognized?"[31] Even if the details of particular individual societies do have a dramatic impact on women's well-being vis-à-vis sex ratios, this point should give us pause, for there is little evidence that unbalanced sex ratios (e.g., in India or China) have generally helped women as a group. Minimally we can say that high sex ratios appear to pose a danger to women's overall social equality, and hence their well-being, even if that danger is not, in every case, realized.

Although such marked preference for boys does not appear to be the case in North America, where sex preferences are split more evenly, there nevertheless exists a documented preference here that *firstborn* children be male. One need only remember an American nursery rhyme to confirm the point:

> First comes love, then comes marriage,
> Then comes [name] with a baby carriage.
> I wish you love, I wish you joy,
> I wish you first a baby boy.
> And when his hair begins to curl,
> I wish you then a baby girl.[32]

Moreover, numerous studies have indicated that firstborn children tend to be more assertive and dominant, and that disproportionate numbers of them hold positions of power and prestige. As a result, feminists tend to fear that widespread sex preselection will bolster gender stereotypes and further impair women's already fragile access to social and economic power.

It is impossible here to resolve whether or not these fears are fully warranted; yet again, it seems at least a strong possibility, even if it is not easily provable.[33] Moreover, insofar as girls *are* chosen to be born second, it seems quite likely that individual daughters will experience negative psychological ramifications in relation to their older brothers, deepening a sense of inferiority already enforced by a patriarchal social structure. As in the previous case, the mere existence of these dangers provides a reason why feminists committed to the principle of equality should treat sex preselection with caution.

Perhaps even more than these worries, however, another concern haunts feminists who consider the matter of sex preselection: sex preselection allows for the symbolic reinforcement of gender inequity. That is, choosing sons is, in a patriarchal society, a choice that fortifies a social bias against females. It functions not simply as a choice, but also as a *symbolic* choice, one that reinforces the social perception that women and girls are less worthy than men and boys. Along these lines, Christine Overall has argued that the choice to preselect boys, while potentially unproblematic in a culture free of misogyny, in our own society functions as a *yes* to patriarchal power.[34] In the judgment of many feminists, even the choice to preselect girls is problematic, since preselecting for sex — *either* sex — necessarily links a child's basic worth to the fact of whether the child is a boy or a girl. Hence, this represents one of the most fundamental ways that we can disrespect a person, while also fortifying social tendencies to link individual worth to gender. Arguing along these lines, Tabitha Powledge has called sex preselection "one of the most stupendously sexist acts in which it is possible to engage . . . the original sexist sin."[35]

Of course, many would deny such a strong assessment. Warren herself admits that this argument against sex selection is among the most troubling. Yet, in her view, the desire to have children of *each* sex — that is, for purposes of family balancing — is not inherently sexist, at least on the surface.[36] Even the choice to opt for male children alone may not be a sexist choice, but rather may be based upon the best interests of the child, for parents may wish that their children be spared the patriarchal restrictions that women still encounter today. This may be especially true in parts of the world where daughters are widely abused and devalued: rather than bring a daughter into the world only to suffer, parents may validly opt for sons instead.

Although it is true that in individual cases sex preselection against girls may reduce female childhood suffering, clearly this is a problematic solution when taken in the aggregate. Trying to remedy patriarchy by eliminating those who suffer under its manifestations — females — is hardly the answer that most people, let alone most feminists, would offer. Moreover, a feminist approach that considers not just the good in individual cases, but also the common good, must consider the social effect that such individual choices have, both on the contours of male-female relations and on the symbolic perception of women in society generally. Social equality between men and women is not well-served by strategies whose cost is the elimination or reduction of large numbers of women, as may be the result in some societies where there is strong male preference. Moreover, such choices, whether they be against female children generally or merely against firstborn females, very likely will further entrench patriarchal attitudes and practices that devalue women, or, at a minimum, will do nothing to challenge those attitudes and practices. Hence, although it may cause no direct harm in individual cases, sex preselection subtly shapes a society in ways inconsonant with feminist commitments to women's flourishing.

The Well-Being of Children

Safety Concerns and the Suffering of Children. Feminist thought clearly must attend carefully to women's well-being, but its concern extends further, to the well-being of all people and indeed to all the earth. Moreover, for reasons outlined above, feminism maintains a special concern for the well-being of children. This is particularly true in the case of the genetic manipulation of offspring, for children as a group are, quite obviously, most directly affected by these technologies; and yet they have minimal ability to speak out, publicly or privately, about whether or not such technologies are justifiably pursued.

From the standpoint of a feminist ethic committed to honoring human embodiment, we must carefully review the impact that technologies of genetic manipulation will have on the physical health and safety of the children concerned. In all three cases of genetic manipulation considered in this book, this impact is largely still unknown. What does seem clear is that there are serious safety concerns with gene therapy as it is currently practiced, and that germ-line gene therapy promises increased risk — risk that may affect not just present but also future generations. Similarly, the risks posed to children born using current methods of sex preselection are still unclear. Hence, although it is impossible accurately to weigh the bodily burden that genetic manipulation will impose upon children, it seems clear that much progress must be made before we can say with any clarity and assurance that physical harm will be minimal.

Yet the physical dangers to children, while very real, must not be allowed to eclipse a critical point: human gene therapy in general has been developed with the clear aim of helping seriously ill children. No feminist approach concerned with children's well-being can afford to overlook this point. The lives of those children who, with the help of these techniques, have found some relief from genetic illness stand as a testimony to the power of genetic manipulation to positively serve human flourishing. To the degree that such techniques could be further developed and applied proactively — that is, to prevent the serious illness from taking hold in the first place — some children will indeed be better off.

Let us probe this point more specifically by turning again to the case studies that we examined earlier. As described in chapter 1, cystic fibrosis (CF) provides a good example of a serious genetic disease for which gene therapy holds much promise. Moreover, should germ-line gene therapy treatment for CF be perfected, no doubt it would represent a vast improvement over current alternative (i.e., drug) therapies, which are unable simultaneously to treat the different organs affected by the disease. Because CF is a serious, indeed life threatening, disease responsible for a great deal of human suffering, and because these alternative treatments have significant drawbacks, genetic manipulation designed to prevent CF, if it could be safely performed, holds a great deal of promise for bettering the lives of many children around the world.

Technologies allowing for sex preselection share some of this promise. Particularly in the case of sex-linked genetic disorders, sex preselection holds forth the possibility that childhood suffering could be prevented, allowing at-risk parents to bear children free of certain genetic diseases (e.g., hemophilia or Duchenne muscular dystrophy). Even in cases where no genetic disease is at stake, sex preselection, as we have noted, may reduce childhood suffering by averting situations where children are born unwanted because they are the "wrong" sex. Feminist thought generally, of course, maintains that insidious social attitudes and practices, not the presence of X and Y chromosomes, are responsible for this gender-based suffering; yet feminists may simultaneously admit that sex preselection could make possible the elimination of some of this suffering (in most cases, suffering by girls), at least in individual cases.[37] Whether or not we should allow or encourage such sex preselection on a broad scale is another matter, particularly when the considerations raised earlier (concerning women's well-being) are taken into account. What seems incontrovertible is that, in some cases, sex preselection, like gene therapy for disease prevention, can indeed function to reduce childhood suffering, even if this result is achieved in a way unacceptable to many feminists.

Ardent supporters of gene therapy argue that childhood suffering likewise may be reduced by genetic manipulation designed to improve memory. Again, most would view a better-than-average memory as a desirable trait, and an obviously deficient memory as an impairment. Moreover, insofar as an excellent memory contributes to general cognitive ability, one can argue that its possession may well improve a child's prospects for overall success and happiness throughout life. Yet most reasonable people stop short of labeling memory enhancement as morally equivalent to disease therapy, except, perhaps, in individuals whose memory is impaired to the point that it interferes dramatically with day-to-day functioning. It seems likely that in many cases memory-enhancement techniques would be aimed not at reducing physical suffering, but rather at giving children an intellectual boost and thus an increased chance of success in the world. This fact makes it more ethically suspect, since enhancing the "normal" is, by most accounts, less pressing than the relief of suffering.[38] Hence, although memory enhancement may in some ways add to children's well-being, the case is not as strong as it is with disease prevention or even sex preselection, when such preselection is specifically designed to reduce suffering.

The Nonobjectification of Children. Genetic manipulation, and perhaps especially memory enhancement, may contradict a feminist ethic in another, less obvious way. A feminist ethic concerned with human flourishing upholds the noninstrumentalization of children as a core value. According to this view, children are not properly viewed as products to be designed according to individual desires, but rather as potentially autonomous beings in their own right, worthy of respect and care for their own sakes. In light of the trends (described in chapter 2) toward viewing children as subject to "quality control," the danger is real that genetic manipulation, particularly in forms that seek to improve upon the "normal," as with the enhancement of an average memory, will further encourage people to consider their children largely as instruments to fulfill their parental desires. Even parents who believe that genetic manipulation would in fact foster a child's own well-being may fail to recognize the ways in which their own individual desires can masquerade under the banner of the child's "best interests," ultimately driving their quest for more "perfect" offspring.

As described above, a major danger here is that parenthood itself will increasingly be conditionalized, so that parents are subtly encouraged to think of their children as made-to-order products that must meet certain individually determined standards of acceptability. Such a view, of course, contradicts the reality that children are never "perfect" and the ideal that parents should accept their children in spite of that fact. Barbara Katz Rothman highlights this danger:

> Parenthood demands . . . total acceptance from us. We expect mothers to love, to accept their babies unreservedly, with the fullness of their hearts, no matter what. We joke about it: "A face only a mother could love. . . . " What does it do to motherhood, to women, and to men as fathers too, when we make parental acceptance conditional, pending further testing? . . . Does the conscious, deliberate emphasis on control and "standards of acceptability" prepare us for the *reality* of parenthood?[39]

Indeed, the idea that parenthood involves, first and foremost, obligation to a child in spite of his or her faults may well be threatened by the view that children's traits are properly and entirely a matter of choice. Some feminist theorists in fact challenge the notion of "choosing" one's children altogether, instead highlighting the fact that parental responsibilities are largely unchosen obligations that we honor even when we find children unattractive or trying.[40] The parent-child bond is marked by a parental fidelity to children regardless of their peculiar characteristics, a sense of obligation that precedes the conscious choices that a parent makes.

Few, of course, would deny that all parents do exercise a certain degree of free choice in shaping their children's lives. Parenting styles have a definite impact on children's abilities and personalities. Yet to extend that control further, encouraging the belief that parents have free control over the "quality" of their (completely malleable) children, simply belies the truth that children are people, not products. Moreover, to focus so heavily on characteristics that may be considered secondary to a child's essential human dignity and basic well-being — characteristics such as beauty, memory, or even gender — conditionalizes parenthood to an extreme degree. As Farley points out in her discussion of sex preselection, "To 'design' our children in terms of their sex, their intelligence or other nonessential characteristics may be to render them acceptable to us not because of their human dignity, not because they are our uniquely gifted children, but only because they fit our pre-conceived desires of what sort of children they must be."[41] Such a move challenges the meaning of procreation generally in a direction that runs counter to the ideal of children's nonobjectification.

In a related vein, the idea that we may completely "design" children according to individual preference plays into and perpetuates the idea that children are akin to private property. The assumption that family bonds are governed by this "ownership" model is extremely problematic from a feminist standpoint, in light of its historic roots in the patriarchal family and, in particular, the ownership by men of women and children. An ownership model of parent-child relationships functions on and encourages an ethic of proprietary control, which traditionally is associated with fathering, rather than a cooperative, supportive, and nurturing parenting style emphasizing growth and preservation, which traditionally is emphasized by mothering.[42] Moreover, such a model moves in the opposite direction from the feminist norm of mutuality, instead valuing dominative power and strong patterns of familial hierarchy. It is a particularly disturbing model of familial relations when considered in light of the high frequency with which child abuse takes place in contemporary U.S. society.

Rather than viewing children as property, a feminist ethic insists that children's well-being is best served by a model of parenting whereby children are supported, nurtured, and encouraged in their development. Although full equality of power and insight between parent and child is not a helpful or even meaningful concept, a feminist parenting style encourages respect for the child as a developing person who someday will be an autonomous individual, and yet who has, and will continue to have, deeply relational instincts and needs as well. Sara Ruddick, in her famed description of "maternal thinking," highlights a parental capacity for "attentive love," a combination of attending, self-restraining, and empathizing whereby a parent may look at and "love a child without seizing or using it, . . . see the child's reality with the patient, loving eye of attention."[43] Such an approach to parenting focuses not on controlling children with a heavy hand, but rather on nurturing their development as persons in their own right. Above all, it disallows the kind of objectification and instrumentalization of a child that is implied by the property analogy.

From the Perspective of Children. To this point I have argued that to treat children as products to be designed or as property to be owned is to *mistreat* them; it is to falsify their reality as dignified persons, resulting in harm to the parent-child relationship and indeed to the notion of parenthood itself. But what of the experience of the children themselves? What exactly would it mean, from a child's point of view, to have been the subject, or potential subject, of genetic manipulation? There is, of course, no one answer to this question. However, feminist philosopher Rosalyn Diprose offers some insight into the question in her discussion of the embodied self as it experiences illness.

Drawing on the thought of Drew Leder, and before him Maurice Merleau-Ponty, Diprose describes the experience of the onset of pain in a man playing tennis who is fully engaged in his game. At first, he does not reflect on his body, and he plays without explicit thought or will. At one point, however, a sudden sharp pain shoots through his body, and immediately he is forced to focus on the well-being (or lack thereof) of his body. As his pain increases, his body becomes the more explicit object of his attention, and he is less able to engage fully with the world or with others; he has experienced a shift in his relation to his body and is now more conscious of it. The body as subject — "dispersed and open to the world prior to the distinctions between mind and body, self and world, self and other" — has become the body as object.[44]

Diprose, again following Merleau-Ponty, holds that this objectification of the body by the self limits one's freedom. Freedom, so understood, is not simply negative freedom from physical and intellectual interference by others; rather, freedom is inherent in the lived body's ability to structure its world and to realize the potentialities informed by its social history. Importantly, other people may challenge and reduce our freedom; they do this by exhibiting an "intolerance of our bodily comportment towards the world, an intolerance which may reduce us from an open-ended mode of belonging to a world to 'being in the world in the way of a thing.'" In other words, others may reduce our freedom by "objectifying our embodied mode of being and so change this to self-reflection."[45] Just as injury functions to objectify the embodied tennis player, causing him to place his body at a distance from his self, the attitudes and actions of others may function to objectify any given person or people, resulting in a similarly disembodied experience and reduction of freedom.

Women, of course, know this all too well. The experience of bodily objectification is constant for many, or even most, women in Western society as they move through a patriarchal world where the sexist attitudes and actions of others — the catcalls, the humiliating advertisements, the unrealistic expectations of body size — demand a level of bodily self-consciousness never experienced by most men. Even when individual women do not face explicitly demeaning experiences, they must function in a society that devalues, degrades, and constantly objectifies the female body. This objectification encourages a sort of bodily alienation and ultimately functions to limit women's freedom.

Let us return to the experience of children, in a world where shaping them genetically is a possibility or even the norm. In such a world it is likely that children will grow up with the knowledge that they are, or are not, genetically designed. A child may know that she was chosen to be a girl, or that her health was ensured by genetic manipulation, or that her memory was enhanced. Or, alternatively, a child may know that he was not genetically manipulated, that his memory is "natural" and perhaps average in comparison to those of his classmates. Some children may not know, and they may wonder: Were they genetically manipulated? Were their (beautiful, intelligent, gregarious) friends?

What effects will such knowledge have on children? It is not unlikely that children who know that they were the subjects of genetic manipulation — for example, for sex selection or memory improvement — will experience various sorts of identity crises or increased levels of parental and social expectation. Feminist philosopher Robyn Rowland voices a common feminist fear that sex-preselected children will carry the burden of their parents' desires and expectations that attach to a particular sex.[46] Similarly, a child with a better-than-average memory may wonder if she is adequately fulfilling the expectations that her parents had when they decided to genetically shape her in the first place. On the other hand, a child who is aware that his parents did not manipulate his genes may worry that he is inadequate to compete with his genetically engineered classmates; indeed, he may find himself in that situation if genetic manipulation becomes so common that nonengineered children are put at a noticeable social or intellectual disadvantage.

The important point here is that a child's knowledge that he or she may or may not be the subject of genetic manipulation may in fact force that child to focus on bodily (or intellectual) strengths and shortcomings in a way that was not previously true. This is the concrete effect of objectification: the child no longer may function relatively unreflectively in the world (like the healthy tennis player), but rather is encouraged to dwell on his or her body as an object, or potential object, of manipulation. The child's self-understanding and self-consciousness have shifted, and now the child is more likely to be in a position of "being in the world in the way of a thing."

There is, of course, no guarantee that any of this will occur. Moreover, the danger of such disembodying, objectifying experiences seems less likely when the genetic manipulation in question is for the prevention of serious disease, because a child "designed" in this way, unlike a child who is sex preselected or whose memory is genetically enhanced, is unlikely to experience added expectations of his or her performance beyond simply living a healthy life.

Yet even if such musings represent only speculation, it is important to pay attention to the dangers that they raise. A feminist ethic concerned not just with individual freedom but also with individual and social well-being cannot afford to ignore or explain away the changes that genetic manipulation may introduce into the lives of children. Furthermore, an ethic that takes seriously our social embeddedness and our bodily existence in the world understands that changes to the genetic makeup of children cannot but have profound effects on the lives of children and of those who care for them.

Social Well-Being: The Socioeconomic Impact of Genetic Manipulation

The final set of issues to be raised under the rubric of feminist thought is the impact that the widespread shaping of offspring is likely to have on our social relations as a whole. In a sense, much of the discussion thus far has already included social relations: relations of women to men, of parents to children, of children to each other and to the broader society. However, there are potential socioeconomic effects of genetic manipulation that do not fall neatly into the categories already described but that deeply impact human well-being. Liberal approaches tend to downplay such socioeconomic considerations in their eagerness to emphasize the freedom of the individual, even at the possible expense of the quality of our common life. The feminist approach put forth here, with its commitment to equitable sharing and human solidarity, challenges this tendency, demanding that we examine the socioeconomic impact of genetic manipulation upon the broad contours of our common life.

To begin with, contemporary feminist commitments to human solidarity issue forth in a call to respect, not erase, human difference. "Difference" is a veritable buzzword of the late twentieth century, as postmodern suspicions of grand narratives have sometimes led academic theorists even to give up on any shared substantive notions of justice or liberation altogether. Yet in spite of multiple problems with the postmodern flight from metanarratives — and, in the arena of ethics, the problems are indeed serious and disturbing[47] — feminism at its best maintains a practical commitment to honor and uphold the value of human diversity and to deal creatively with differences. This includes, minimally, differences of race, gender, and class, but it also may be understood to extend outward to differences of intelligence, body type, and so on.

Hence, a feminist commitment to diversity includes the recognition that there is no one "perfect" human body. Rather, a diversity of bodies and body types exists in the world, and that diversity generally is of positive value. Indeed, the modern history of eugenics, coupled with persistent racial, ethnic, and gender discrimination, should make us wary of any move that encourages the valuation of certain body types over others without good reason. It must be recognized that popular images of the "perfect" human body are necessarily malleable, the product of social construction. Who, finally, determines what is "perfect"? Barbara Katz Rothman addresses this issue in the context of prenatal diagnosis, arguing that the social ideologies of patriarchy and capitalism shape our understanding of, and desire for, human perfection:

> What constitutes perfection . . . ? Who, if not the creators of the square tomato, the efficient but painfully distended milk-producing cow, are going to set the standards of perfection? Perfection is *for* something. The perfect tomato is perfectly marketable. And the perfect child?[48]

Because our standards of perfection are so influenced by the social context in which we live, and because that social context is one that includes a marked hostility toward women (and, it may be added, persons socially disempowered for other reasons), feminists in particular have reason to raise a note of caution about technologies that encourage us to seek "perfection" in our offspring.

The danger is particularly acute in the case of genetic enhancement: individual preferences about the kinds of enhancements to be made would, no doubt, reflect ephemeral social preference and could place an added strain on race and gender relations. Such social preferences generally tend to reinforce an iniquitous status quo, because "given that all too many people will want their children to fit prevailing social norms, even when these norms happen to be sexist, racist, and classist in nature, gene therapy for enhancement purposes will only make the struggle for equity between men and women that much more difficult."[49] Extending the analysis to include race, it seems at least possible that widespread "enhancement" manipulations — including, for instance, efforts to lighten skin tone in order to ease a child's social acceptance — could function to exacerbate insidious racial tension and discrimination. Insofar as genetic manipulation does this, it works directly against the goals of inclusivity and acceptance of human diversity.

Some theorists take a step further the idea that our images of the "perfect" body reflect transitory social preferences; they argue that the categories of illness and disease are themselves purely the product of social construction. Hence, focusing on technological solutions to genetic disease is a wrongheaded emphasis, for it ignores the crux of the problem (i.e., society's lack of accommodation to different bodily abilities) and simultaneously devalues the lives of those currently living with such disease. According to an extreme version of this view, honoring human diversity includes a commitment to resisting all forms of gene therapy, even those seeking to prevent serious genetic illness. Instead of pouring resources into gene therapy, thereby augmenting a social bias against the disabled, we should attempt to change society's level of acceptance of, and accommodation to, genetic disability.

I do not wish to adopt this more extreme line of argumentation, although surely it is true that we, as individuals and as a society, would do well to reevaluate our understanding of what constitutes "disability," including the ways that we can make our world more hospitable to persons with physical or mental impairments.[50] Yet even if the line demarcating health from disease (and, by extension, "normal" from "abnormal" states of the body) is somewhat fuzzy, I do not believe that it is so malleable that we may effectively do away with it altogether. Most reasonable persons agree that "serious" genetic illness constitutes disease, an abnormal and undesirable state of affairs that should be eliminated if safe means are available to do so. Moreover, seeking to prevent genetic disease need not imply a devaluation of the lives of those currently living with such disease; as Rosemarie Tong points out, addressing the case of Down syndrome, "The fact that a child or adult with Down syndrome can lead a productive and happy life does not mean that the same child or adult would turn down the opportunity to lead an even more productive and happy life — that is, a life not bound by the limitations that Down syndrome imposes on its subjects."[51] In other words, it *is* possible to make important judgment calls about the desirability of genetic diseases based on the well-being of those who live with them. Indeed, it is part of what an ethic committed to human flourishing must do.

Nevertheless, it is wise to remain alert to the danger that genetic technologies may be used not to relieve human suffering, but rather to eliminate human diversity. Indeed, when, exactly, is a condition worthy of genetic "treatment"? Otherwise put, when is diversity a desirable thing, and when does it represent harmful deviation from a state of health and normalcy? Moreover, who, in the end, will decide which genetic conditions are properly treated? In light of the painful history of eugenics outlined in chapter 2, we must insist on caution in this regard. Any lines that are drawn to demarcate the "normal" from the "abnormal" (with the latter trait a proper object of genetic manipulation) must be justified with a concept of well-being in mind *that includes* a strong commitment to upholding human diversity.

Related to concerns about diversity, feminists worry about the effect that genetic manipulation is likely to have on existing socioeconomic tensions. It seems probable that the cost of genetically manipulating offspring will be high, so that only relatively advantaged women or couples will be able to afford it. Hence, these genetic technologies have the potential dramatically to exacerbate socioeconomic inequality. Again, if gene therapy gains widespread acceptance and use, then genetic diseases such as cystic fibrosis very likely will become a class-stratified phenomenon, with those who are economically well-off being able to purchase their way out.

The issue of justice in regard to the distribution of healthcare is, of course, a complicated one, deserving more space than is possible here. Yet minimally we can say that the unwillingness on the part of many liberals to weigh seriously the socioeconomic effects of genetic manipulation is disturbing. For its part, a feminist commitment to equitable sharing demands that the distribution of any facet of healthcare provision, including genetic manipulation, not contribute further to a vast and ever widening gap (in the United States and worldwide) between the rich and the poor. If genetic manipulation is to be allowed or encouraged, it must be done in such a way that it will benefit not only the relatively well-off socioeconomic classes; its gains must be felt by all.

Beyond equitable distribution, a further concern surfaces about the justness of using scarce medical resources to support the infrastructure necessary to develop and implement genetic manipulation. When forty-one million people in the United States lack insurance for even the most basic forms of healthcare, how can such high-tech procedures, benefiting a relatively small number of people, be justified?[52] Along these lines, our Western propensity to overemphasize technological solutions to problems may in fact distract us from more "mundane" issues such as the organization of healthcare generally. Similarly, a focus on genetic manipulation may well turn us away from crucial environmental (non-genetic) factors that also contribute heavily to human disease; in fact, it may be that "our problems lie in darker corners, in poverty and the poor nutrition and inadequate healthcare and increasing homelessness that accompany poverty in America."[53] In this light, it may be not only unfair but also imprudent to devote scarce healthcare dollars to the infrastructure necessary to support genetic manipulation, since money may be better spent elsewhere, from a strictly cost-benefit point of view.

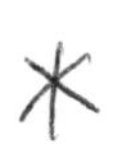

Critics of such egalitarian approaches argue that, in a capitalist economy, it is wrong to prevent those with sufficient resources to purchase whatever forms of healthcare they desire. Yet it must be reiterated that the expenses associated with genetic manipulation are not simply those borne by individuals who wish to make use of the technology; rather, they include vast amounts of resources, public and private, currently devoted to the research and development of the technologies. Again, it is impossible to resolve, or even to do justice to, this complicated topic here. Nevertheless, a feminist approach minimally must raise a challenge to this expenditure of resources, which seems, at least on the surface, to fly in the face of social well-being by privileging high-tech solutions for the few over low-tech aid to the many.

From Procreative Liberty to Human Well-Being as a Feminist Norm

The foregoing considerations raise serious questions about whether we as a society or as individuals should actively pursue genetic technologies for manipulating offspring traits. I have argued that an adequate feminist perspective—that is, one that seeks a holistic vision for the well-being of persons, including both their autonomy and their embodied relationality—necessarily challenges accounts that privilege procreative liberty exclusively and thus place almost no limits on genetic manipulation. That said, I do not mean to imply that we must abandon genetic manipulation outright because it threatens to harm women, objectify and instrumentalize children, and damage the common good. Rather, the task is to identify *which* forms of genetic manipulation truly enhance human well-being—that is, which are really in children's best interests and will be least likely to lead to the dangers described above.

Put another way, a feminist analysis that upholds both autonomy and embodied relationality as components of human well-being cannot afford to ignore either. Hence, it insists that the choice for genetic manipulation must be one grounded not purely in procreative liberty, but rather in the well-being of persons understood as embodied, socially embedded, integral human beings. It is this more comprehensive vision of human well-being that constitutes feminism's most incisive contribution to an ethical evaluation of genetic manipulation.

Notes

1. Mary Midgley and Judith Hughes, *Women's Choices: Philosophical Problems Facing Feminism* (London: Weidenfeld & Nicolson, 1983), 223–24.

2. Here I am using the term "liberal" not in the contemporary political sense, but rather in the classic sense of liberal philosophical thought — that is, thought that privileges the value of individual liberty.

3. John Robertson, *Children of Choice: Freedom and the New Reproductive Technologies* (Princeton, N. J.: Princeton University Press, 1994), 16.

4. Ibid., 430.

5. John A. Robertson, "Genetic Selection of Offspring Characteristics," *Boston University Law Review* 76, no. 3 (1996): 466–68.

6. Ibid., 465. Robertson seems to equivocate a bit over the course of his writings about whether to protect nontherapeutic enhancement under the mantle of procreative liberty. In certain places he appears to be more concerned to protect the right to have healthy offspring and less enthusiastic about enhancing offspring characteristics. Yet he does not prohibit the latter, and in later writings he appears to support genetic enhancement squarely under the scope of procreative liberty. See Robertson, *Children of Choice,* 263 n. 40, 166–67; "Procreative Liberty and the Control of Conception, Pregnancy, and Childbirth," *Virginia Law Review* 69, no. 3 (1983): 432; "Genetic Selection of Offspring Characteristics," 436–37.

7. Notably, Robertson insists that a given practice does no "harm" to a child if that child would never have been born without the practice in question. If the child would not be born at all without the technique in question, there are no grounds for ceasing the technique, even if it leads to all but the most debilitating birth defects and the like. This is how he justifies the intentional diminishment of offspring. See Robertson, "Procreative Liberty and the State's Burden of Proof in Regulating Noncoital Reproduction," *Law, Medicine, and Health Care* 16, nos. 1–2 (1988): 20–21; "Embryos, Families, and Procreative Liberty: The Legal Structure of the New Reproduction," *Southern California Law Review* 59 (1986): 987; "In Vitro Conception and Harm to the Unborn," *Hastings Center Report* 8, no. 5 (1978): 14.

8. Robertson, *Children of Choice,* 227.

9. Mary Ann Warren, *Gendercide: The Implications of Sex Selection* (Totowa, N.J.: Rowman & Allanheld, 1985).

10. Elizabeth A. Johnson, *She Who Is: The Mystery of God in Feminist Theological Discourse* (New York: Crossroad, 1992), 63, 30–31; see also Rosemary Radford Ruether, *Sexism and God-Talk: Toward a Feminist Theology* (Boston: Beacon Press, 1983), 18–19.

11. Feminism, at its best, is concerned more broadly, of course, with the well-being of *all* persons (women, men, and children), and indeed with the well-being of all the earth. Since contemporary feminism takes as axiomatic the existence of patriarchy, however, it aims to "correct this bias by a bias for women" (Margaret A. Farley, "Feminist Ethics," in *The Westminster Dictionary of Christian Ethics,* ed. James F. Childress and John Macquarrie [Philadelphia: Westminster, 1986], 229).

12. Beverly Wildung Harrison, *Our Right to Choose: Toward a New Ethic of Abortion* (Boston: Beacon Press, 1983), 4, 38.

13. Barbara Ehrenreich and Deirdre English, *For Her Own Good: 150 Years of the Experts' Advice to Women* (New York: Doubleday, 1978).

14. Ibid., 43–44, 45–46.

15. Radical feminism, as a category within feminism generally, is quite broad and can be difficult to specify. Generally we can say that radical feminists believe that distinctions based on gender lie at the heart of human experience and that patriarchy is the most basic form of human oppression. Radical feminists generally move beyond liberal feminism's emphasis on the individual liberty of women and instead call for the elimination of patriarchy more broadly in its physical, psychological, and cultural dimensions. Often the line is blurred between so-called radical feminism and socialist feminism, which more readily includes economic dimensions in its analysis of oppression. See Alison M. Jaggar, *Feminist Politics and Human Nature* (Totowa, N.J.: Rowman & Allanheld, 1983); Margaret A. Farley, "Feminism and Universal Morality," in *Prospects for a Common Morality,* ed. Gene Outka and John P. Reeder Jr. (Princeton, N.J.: Princeton University Press, 1993), 174–77.

16. Barbara Katz Rothman, "The Meanings of Choice in Reproductive Technology," in *Test Tube Women: What Future for Motherhood?* ed. Rita Arditti, Renate Duelli Klein, and Shelley Minden (Boston: Pandora Press, 1984), 32; Rothman quotes Ruth Hubbard, 27.

17. Barbara Katz Rothman, "The Products of Conception: The Social Context of Reproductive Choices," *Journal of Medical Ethics* 11 (1985): 191–92.

18. Margaret A. Farley, "Feminist Theology and Bioethics," in *Women's Consciousness, Women's Conscience,* ed. Barbara Hilkert Andolsen, Christine E. Gudorf, and Mary D. Pellauer (San Francisco: Harper & Row, 1985), 292–93.

19. Barbara Katz Rothman, *Recreating Motherhood: Ideology and Technology in a Patriarchal Society* (New York: W. W. Norton, 1989), 249.

20. Ibid., 58.

21. Farley, "Feminism and Universal Morality," 182.

22. Johnson, *She Who Is,* 68.

23. Maura A. Ryan, "Justice and Artificial Reproduction: A Catholic Feminist Analysis" (Ph.D. diss., Yale University, 1993), 43; see also Beverly Wildung Harrison, *Making the Connections: Essays in Feminist Social Ethics* (Boston: Beacon Press, 1985), 253.

24. Margaret A. Farley, "New Patterns of Relationship: Beginnings of a Moral Revolution," *Theological Studies* 36 (1975): 632; Barbara Hilkert Andolsen, "Agape in Feminist Theological Ethics," in *Feminist Theological Ethics: A Reader,* ed. Lois K. Daly (Louisville: Westminster John Knox, 1994), 154; see also Margaret A. Farley, *Personal Commitments: Beginning, Keeping, Changing* (San Francisco: Harper & Row, 1986), chapter 7; Harrison, *Making the Connections,* 18–19; Christine E. Gudorf, "Parenting, Mutual Love, and Sacrifice," in Andolsen, Gudorf, and Pellauer, eds., *Women's Consciousness, Women's Conscience,* 175–91.

25. Shelley Minden, "Patriarchal Designs: The Genetic Engineering of Human Embryos," in *Made to Order: The Myth of Reproductive and Genetic Progress,* ed. Patricia Spallone and Deborah Lynn Steinberg (New York: Pergamon Press, 1987), 102.

26. Robyn Rowland, "Of Women Born, But for How Long? The Relationship of Women to the New Reproductive Technologies and the Issue of Choice," in Spallone and Steinberg, eds., *Made to Order,* 77.

27. Lisa Sowle Cahill, *Sex, Gender, and Christian Ethics* (Cambridge: Cambridge University Press, 1996), 245.

28. Rothman, *Recreating Motherhood*, 19.

29. Maura A. Ryan, "The Argument for Unlimited Procreative Liberty: A Feminist Critique," *Hastings Center Report* 20, no. 4 (1990): 12.

30. Warren, *Gendercide*, 135–37; see also Robyn Rowland, "Motherhood, Patriarchal Power, Alienation and the Issue of 'Choice' in Sex Preselection," in *Man-Made Women: How New Reproductive Technologies Affect Women*, ed. Gena Corea et al. (London: Hutchinson, 1985), 81, citing Marcia Guttentag and Paul F. Secord, *Too Many Women? The Sex Ratio Question* (Beverly Hills, Calif.: Sage, 1983), 231.

31. Rowland, "Motherhood," 83. Robertson, by contrast, uncritically puts forth the suggestion that a high sex ratio, and thus a "shortage" of women, will likely lead to a scenario whereby women's social value (and presumably their well-being) will actually be "bid up" according to "market" forces, in keeping with women's relative scarcity. The idea here is that "nature," or market forces, or whatever one chooses to call it, will correct for skewed sex ratios, eventually making it seem more profitable for parents to choose to have girls rather than boys, correcting the imbalance. See Robertson, "Genetic Selection of Offspring Characteristics," 458; also J. Egozcue, "Sex Selection: Why Not?" *Human Reproduction* 8, no. 11 (1993): 1777. Although this argument is put forth in the literature with some regularity, I cannot find any evidence cited that would suggest that such a happy result has occurred, or is likely to occur, in existing societies with high sex ratios.

32. Quoted in Roberta Steinbacher and Helen B. Holmes, "Sex Choice: Survival and Sisterhood," in Corea et al., eds., *Man-Made Women*, 52.

33. Warren, for her part, again challenges such fears, arguing that the studies done are unclear and that they fail to resolve crucial methodological problems concerning the isolation of birth order from other factors such as family size and socioeconomic status. Hence, she does not believe that the evidence supports the seemingly obvious judgment that firstborns are more apt to be high achievers, nor does she believe that girls and women as a whole will necessarily be harmed if they are more often chosen to be second-born. See Warren, *Gendercide*, 138–42.

34. Christine Overall, *Ethics and Human Reproduction: A Feminist Analysis* (Boston: Allen & Unwin, 1987), 21–28.

35. Tabitha M. Powledge, "Unnatural Selection: On Choosing Children's Sex," in *The Custom-Made Child? Women-Centered Perspectives*, ed. Helen B. Holmes, Betty B. Hoskins, and Michael Gross (Clifton, N.J.: Humana Press, 1981), 196.

36. Warren, *Gendercide*, 83–88. Warren does acknowledge, however, that the choice for family balancing of sex may depend on underlying assumptions that are themselves sexist. For instance, a father of two girls may wish for a son with whom to go fishing and play ball — activities that presumably girls also could enjoy. Hence, gender stereotyping may wrongly contribute to the perception that family balance, in terms of gender, is a valid reason for sex selection. It is important to note that harmful gender stereotyping may in fact be aggravated by the practice of sex preselection, since parents will be encouraged to develop gendered images of their children's personalities even before birth.

37. I do not mean to imply here that there is an exact parallel to be drawn between sexist social attitudes and structures, on the one hand, and a social structure that makes it difficult to live with serious genetic illness, on the other. Some have made this argument, highlighting the social construction of disease and thereby holding that we should focus not on developing gene therapy treatments, but rather on making the world a more welcoming place for women *and* for those with genetic illness or disabilities. While not rejecting this approach entirely, I do find a difference between the prevention of serious disease and the prevention of being female, thereby being subject to the suffering associated with patriarchy. That is, in my view, serious illness necessarily contradicts human flourishing in a way that being female does not.

38. As discussed above, defining what qualifies as "normal" is a difficult task, since the interpretation of the term itself is heavily influenced by prevailing social structures and cultural practices. From one perspective, the sociocultural constructedness of what is considered normal in fact highlights why enhancing so-called normal characteristics is indeed less pressing than relieving serious disease.

39. Rothman, "Products of Conception," 190.

40. Ryan, "Argument for Unlimited Procreative Liberty," 10.

41. Margaret A. Farley, "Selecting Your Baby's Sex: Beware of Social Abuses," *New York Daily News*, October 11, 1998, 59; see also Ryan, "Argument for Unlimited Procreative Liberty," 8.

42. Janet Farrell Smith, "Parenting and Property," in *Mothering: Essays in Feminist Theory*, ed. Joyce Trebilcot (Totowa, N.J.: Rowman & Allanheld, 1983), 201, 206, 208; see also Cahill, *Sex, Gender, and Christian Ethics*, 243.

43. Sara Ruddick, "Maternal Thinking," in Trebilcot, ed., *Mothering*, 224.

44. Rosalyn Diprose, *The Bodies of Women: Ethics, Embodiment and Sexual Difference* (London and New York: Routledge, 1994), 104.

45. Ibid., 107.

46. Rowland, "Motherhood," 84.

47. These problems become especially apparent when "difference" is upheld not as a practical consideration, but rather as a philosophical principle. For an excellent critical analysis of the problems associated with a postmodern approach in the realm of ethics see Cahill, *Sex, Gender, and Christian Ethics*, esp. 25–30.

48. Barbara Katz Rothman, "Of Maps and Imaginations: Sociology Confronts the Genome," *Social Problems* 42, no. 1 (1995): 8.

49. Rosemarie Tong, *Feminist Approaches to Bioethics: Theoretical Reflections and Practical Applications* (Boulder, Colo.: Westview Press, 1997), 241.

50. In contrast to more extreme views, Adrienne Asch provides a helpful and relatively nonideological articulation of the point that disease is, in large part, socially constructed, and therefore we should not simply seek to eliminate disability, but rather should alter the ways in which we think about it. In her view, we should frame our understanding of disability by an acknowledgment of our hopes and dreams vis-à-vis the experience of raising children, asking ourselves whether and how those hopes and dreams would be compromised by a child's disability. This sort of discussion would allow us to identify the ways in which society could be changed to be more welcoming to disabled children, rather than automatically to frame disabled children themselves as the problem. Here Asch does not address gene therapy, but rather the phenomenon of

prenatal diagnosis and selective abortion. See Adrienne Asch, "Reproductive Technology and Disability," in *Reproductive Laws for the 1990s,* ed. Sherill Cohen and Nadine Taub (Clifton, N.J.: Humana Press, 1989), esp. 84–86.

51. Tong, *Feminist Approaches to Bioethics,* 239.

52. As Leroy Walters and Julie Gage Palmer point out, individual genetic diseases can be rare, but collectively they are responsible for a great deal of suffering. See LeRoy Walters and Julie Gage Palmer, *The Ethics of Human Gene Therapy* (New York: Oxford University Press, 1997), 15.

53. Barbara Katz Rothman, "Not All That Glitters Is Gold," *Hastings Center Report* 22, no. 4, special supplement, "Genetic Grammar" (1992): S14.

Chapter Four

On God and Giftedness

Christian Approaches to "Designing" Children

IN 1931 Reformed scholar Georgia Harkness used these words to describe Christian reformer John Calvin's conviction about human procreation: "God makes the grass to grow; God fecundates the beasts; God gives human progeny. Fertility, like continence, is the gift of God."[1] This sort of confidence that God plays the central role in the procreative process undeniably has eroded in a modern, increasingly secular age. Moreover, the advent of technological birth control means that today human beings *do* have an unprecedented degree of control over their fertility. Indeed, liberal theorist John Robertson's words illustrate how far a typically modern understanding about the divine role in procreation is from that of Calvin: "The decision to have or not have children is, at some important level, no longer a matter of God or nature, but has been made subject to human will and technical expertise."[2] Nevertheless, even as millions of persons the world over, including Christians, make use of various technological means for controlling whether and when they have children, the Christian tradition continues to bequeath the recognition that on some level God is profoundly present in the mystery of procreation, and that God's very presence matters somehow in determining how human beings should approach the process of having children, including the ways in which they should, or should not, manipulate their children's genetic profiles.

The purpose of this chapter is to probe some of the central insights that the Christian tradition offers that bear upon the issue of genetic manipulation, particularly the genetic manipulation of offspring.

Specifically, I will examine three key themes generally present within contemporary Christianity:[3] (1) the understanding that children are to be viewed as gifts from God and that parenthood itself is a vocation ordered under God; (2) the claim that human beings are called to intervene responsibly in nature; and (3) the affirmation of the common good as a positive value by which to evaluate moral activity. Taken together, these three themes begin to point toward a positive vision for evaluating the genetic manipulation of children. Furthermore, although some of these themes partially overlap with feminist insights, it is my belief that the Christian tradition offers a unique wisdom — wisdom that not only supplements previously articulated feminist insights regarding human well-being, but also opens the way forward to a deeper understanding of what that human well-being might entail with respect to our relations with God and with each other.

Having Children in Christian Perspective

The Vocation of Parenthood

Whatever else modern Western society has to say about human procreation, it assuredly upholds the idea that parenthood is above all a matter of individual choice. The advent of modern forms of birth control means that we may to a large extent choose if and when we will have children; and, within certain socially prescribed limits, parents are relatively free to raise their children as they see fit. Moreover, as discussed in earlier chapters of this work, a disturbing increase in the desire for "perfect" children indicates a heightened sense of control that potential parents today have over the characteristics of their progeny.

Although some Christian thinkers have upheld the desirability of a purely choice-oriented model of parenthood, it is fair to characterize the tradition as a whole as raising up an alternate vision, one that places sharper limits on human choice and simultaneously more closely connects the experience of parenthood with one's life before God. Perhaps the most pivotal historical figure in this regard is Martin Luther. Earlier prominent Christian theologians, such as Augustine and Thomas

Aquinas, very often discussed offspring in the context of their belief that procreation, while good and necessary for species preservation, also functioned in part to justify otherwise sinful sexual relations that are themselves a part of the lesser institution of marriage (in contrast to the higher good of celibacy). In contrast, Luther portrayed marriage and procreation themselves as part of a holy vocation, one instituted by God and whose function is to serve and honor God. Thus, having children, in Luther's view, is above all a context in which God meets us and in which we live out our faith; he refers to it as "in all the world . . . the noblest and most precious work."[4] Luther speaks freely about the wonders of pregnancy, childbirth, and childrearing, and he urges fathers and mothers alike to engage in the mundane tasks of childcare with a spirit of joy and trust and an attitude of faithfulness to God.

In short, parenthood, according to Luther, is not simply a matter of the individual's choice to have children; rather, it is a holy vocation ordered under the divine will. Furthermore, the manner in which parents raise their children is not to be dictated merely by parental preference; parents are mandated to bear children for their own sake and to bring them up in the godly life. We may want to debate Luther about what this concretely entails for parents — Luther does indeed uphold certain practices in childrearing that would be deeply disturbing to many parents in contemporary times — but the crucial point for the present discussion is that, for Luther, having children fits into a larger scheme of God's will for human persons. As such, it is deeply interrelated with Christian convictions about how we are to live life under God.

The theme of parenthood as vocation is echoed clearly in much of contemporary theology. For instance, ethicist Karen Lebacqz, examining parenthood in scriptural perspective, draws on the stories of Abraham and Sarah and of Job to illustrate how parenthood should be understood as a way of responding to God's call — that is, a vocation. Similarly, James Gustafson argues that marriage and family are a calling in service to God's ordering and caring for the world. In other words, marriage is not simply an individual covenant; rather, it serves broader values, values having to do with God's ordering of the universe.[5] In each of these cases parenthood itself is set within the broader context of faithfulness to God, who has purposes for humankind.

Although choice is not here excluded from the process of procreation, it is simply not the defining mark of what it means to be a parent. Ethicist Maura Ryan, challenging the notion that we are free to choose all obligations, highlights the "givenness" and duration of parental responsibilities; kinship connections invoke a transcendent commitment that remains, even when persons seem unattractive to us. She writes,

> The common expression, "This child has a face only a mother could love" speaks . . . about acceptance and fidelity to children, even to those whose looks or gender or genetic characteristics are not what the parent would have desired or what meets society's standards. We have accepted the fact that, unlike a product in the market, children cannot be returned or exchanged if found to be other than what was expected.[6]

According to this view, the moral life cannot be reduced to chosen relationships, and nowhere is this more true than in the process of having and raising children. Again, this does not mean that a Christian view of parenthood should remove choice altogether from the procreative process. Rather, choice simply does not, indeed cannot, tell the whole story of what it *means* to be a parent. That is, when we highlight choice at the expense of all other values, we lose touch with a critical part of the experience of parenting under God.

Children as Gifts

If parenthood is understood as a vocation ordered under the divine will, how shall we view children? In sharp contrast to the idea that adults have a personal "right" to have (or not to have) children, the Christian tradition in general has upheld the idea that children are best understood not as rights, but as gifts for whom we are to be grateful to God. Parents may have responsibilities to nurture and foster the development of the children who are entrusted to them, but these same children, like all persons, "belong" to God. Hence, like the rest of us, children possess a dignity and a "poetry" that commands an attitude of respectful awe.[7] They are not properly objects of ownership or domination.

The roots of this understanding of children as dignified and valuable in and of themselves lie both in the theologies of creation and incarnation and in the ministry of Jesus. According to the general Christian understanding of creation, God made human beings, male and female, in God's image and pronounced them to be "good." Although there is some diversity in Christian thought about how best to interpret human responsibility under this doctrine of creation, there is general agreement that creation in God's image lends a dignity to all human persons that we are obligated to respect. This dignity is further supported by the doctrine of the incarnation, whereby God so loves the world that God, in the person of Jesus Christ, has defined the divine self as somehow inclusive of the human. Finally, Jesus' ministry supports the idea that all human beings are valuable in and of themselves; Jesus himself taught, in word and deed, that each person is loved by God and that we in turn are to love one another. Moreover, Jesus gathered children around him and often spoke of the special relation of children to God's kingdom, implying in part that children deserve special concern and protection as *God's* children.

The Christian sacrament of child/infant baptism signifies the understanding that children are utterly valuable to God, and that indeed they belong first to God and are entrusted only secondarily to their parents. In baptism, parents symbolically hand the child over to God, communicating that there are limits to the "nurture" that they can and should provide.[8] This means that on some level parental desires for a child need to be relinquished, for while it is appropriate for parents to exercise responsibility for the care and upbringing of their children, those children are not to be understood simply as objects for their parents to mold.

Hence, this Christian recognition of the giftedness of children seems to support, among other things, not seeking absolute control over every aspect of a child's being, including his or her genetic makeup. Genetic manipulation intensifies the already present danger of objectifying the human subject, of seeing a child as something less than the mysterious, whole, unique person that he or she is, and viewing a child instead as an object to be designed in accordance with some individual or social purpose. In the words of one bioethicist, "There is a danger that we may lose the sense of a child as a gift and come to look upon children as means to an end, an end that is as carefully designed and programmed as possible."[9] Rather than viewing children as objects of parental desire and genetic control, then, Christianity exhorts parents and others to respect children as fully dignified, albeit not yet fully autonomous, members of the human community, lovable in and of themselves and not for their ability to meet parental aspirations or to fulfill particular parental desires.

It is, of course, possible to urge respect and nonobjectification of children without going so far as to condemn all forms of technological reproduction and genetic manipulation. Rather than assuming too quickly that technical intervention destroys in parents a proper sense of awe and respect before their children, we must examine particular technologies and determine whether or not they may lead us to objectify children, to treat or even to view them inappropriately or in ways contrary to their well-being. Christian faith leads us to understand the lives of children as valuable, dignified, and worthy of care and respect. Any given form of genetic manipulation must not violate or threaten this reality.

Christian ethicist Stanley Hauerwas has written extensively and eloquently on the Christian understanding of children as gifts. Hauerwas argues vehemently against the liberal assumption that we "choose" our children, maintaining, "If the language of choice is to be used at all in describing our willingness to have children it must be qualified and controlled by the more fundamental metaphor of gift."[10] He argues that the idea that we must *choose* our children leads us to place an unrealistic demand on them to be perfect; moreover, it also causes parents to feel overly responsible for children's well-being, blaming themselves when, for instance, children inherit a "baldness" gene, or when they cannot offer round-the-clock, nonstop attention to a child's development. Against this background, he argues, it is understandable that more and more people decide against having children altogether, perceiving it as too great a moral burden.

It is in children with retardation that Hauerwas identifies a particularly intense form of the giftedness of children. According to his view, persons with retardation, by virtue of their difference, help the Christian community to understand crucial aspects of what it means to be a diverse community in the first place. Hence, besides bringing their own special gifts and joys, even by way of their limits they enrich the Christian community and encourage us to accept human frailty. Furthermore, persons with retardation provide their parents with the means to help them "break through the myths and illusions that our social order wants us to accept — namely, that life is about being members of the 'Pepsi generation.' "[11] By their very presence they encourage us to trust our better judgment, in a way that "perfect" children cannot do.

Hence, in Hauerwas's view, our task is not to seek a high degree of control over, and responsibility for, the "quality" of our children. Rather, Christians should view children as an occasion to love those whom we do not necessarily "choose" to love, to "love them for what they are rather than what we want or wish them to be."[12] This is, in fact, part of the nature of their giftedness; children draw our love even while refusing to conform to our expectations. In Hauerwas's analysis, nonmanipulative love — that is, unconditional love — is based on regard for another who is not under one's control.

Respecting and Loving Our Children

Hauerwas is not alone in his emphasis on nonmanipulative love as the appropriate response to the gift of children. Christian ethicists generally have striven to emphasize that children demand both our respect and our unconditional love. Such love places limits on the desire to shape and transform other human beings as if they were infinitely malleable. This does not mean that parents should not nurture their children's growth and development; rather, such parental nurture should take place in the context of a basic acceptance of children in all their frailty, weakness, and imperfection. Gilbert Meilaender argues the point:

> In our saner moments we know that parents today are far too eager to use the methods already available — chiefly in the realm of controlling nurture rather than nature — to shape the lives of their children. We are unwilling to let the mystery of personhood — equal in dignity to our own — unfold in the lives of our children. . . . The nurture of children sometimes should be demanding, but . . . [we should] seek to shape and nurture only those whom we first accept without qualification.[13]

In fact, according to the Christian understanding, unconditional love seems to demand such acceptance, because that is how God loves human beings: in the midst of their faults and failings.

Many have raised a note of caution about how the phenomenon of genetic manipulation may alter our propensity to offer such respect, love, and acceptance. The World Council of Churches, for instance, in its document *Manipulating Life,* maintains that viewing humanity as an object of genetic manipulation reduces the mutual respect among persons that Christians should strive to foster.[14] Moral theologian Richard McCormick focuses more specifically on the love that we should offer individual children; he warns that preferential breeding in general may begin to pervert our attitudes: "I believe it is naive to think that we can program for certain characteristics and continue for long to 'love the child for itself' when it does not have them."[15] The fear here is that a society that thinks of children as something at its disposal, something to be made according to individual wishes, will be unable to continue to love and respect children as they should be loved and respected. That is, a gradual shift in social practices in this regard may in fact precipitate a change in our individual and collective beliefs. Theologian Oliver O'Donovan articulates the point succinctly: "When we start making human beings we necessarily stop loving them."[16]

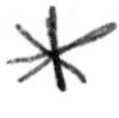

It certainly is true that thinking of children, even subconsciously, as primarily a means to achieving parental satisfaction undermines the call to respect them, let alone to love them unconditionally. Yet again, one might pose the question whether this is *necessarily* the case with every form of reproductive and genetic technology. It seems conceivable, even likely, that certain forms of genetic manipulation, for instance, do not conduce to an attitude of molding or "making" children, but rather may be viewed as a form of helping, even loving them.

After all, helping children who suffer can hardly be classified as harmful; part of the central mission of Jesus himself was to heal the sick. The United Church of Christ, in its 1989 pronouncement on the church and genetic engineering, proclaimed strongly that followers of Jesus are called to carry on his healing work. Along similar lines, ethicist Allen Verhey points out the Christian tradition's belief that God's cause is life and human flourishing, including health, not disease.[17] Love of neighbor surely demands at least *some* willingness to intervene, even genetically, on behalf of human health. Moreover, although the line between disease prevention and enhancement may be difficult to draw, a strong segment of the tradition holds that this line is important nevertheless.

Yet in spite of the exhortation to heal the sick and relieve human suffering, even suffering itself is a slippery concept. The theological insight that suffering may in some way teach or transform us complicates any straightforward interpretation that suffering is the absolute enemy of human dignity. Suffering surely is a context for God's mercy in the form of healing and support. Yet Christians also point out that suffering itself functions to remind us of life's fragility. Stanley Hauerwas, for instance, argues that too often we seek to eliminate, rather than care for, those who cause us discomfort — for example, mentally disabled persons. Hauerwas believes that we are called to prevent unnecessary suffering (including preventable retardation), but he cautions against the idea that we should *always* seek to prevent suffering. "In the very attempt to escape suffering," he asks, "do we not lose something of our own humanity? . . . We are never quite what we should be until we recognize the necessity and inevitability of suffering in our lives."[18]

All of this suggests that Christian tradition calls people to discern the balance between acting to relieve human suffering and yet realizing that there are important limits as to what we can, and should, do to eliminate it. Certainly the history of eugenics reminds us of the dangers that can result when the instinct to relieve human suffering and "improve" the human situation recognizes no limits. Here it is important simply to note that neighbor-love for children entails a complex mixture of positive action to promote their health and well-being, on the one hand, and an open-armed acceptance of their all-too-human frailties, on the other. Moreover, although we are obligated to show our love to children by preventing their suffering, perhaps even by using tools of genetic manipulation, *no* technological intervention should threaten both the respect and the unconditional love that all children, including those who are less than "perfect," are due.

Responsible Intervention in Nature

The second general Christian theme worthy of examination is the idea that human beings are called by God to intervene responsibly in nature. Responsible intervention is not unlimited intervention; rather, Christianity recognizes limits appropriate to the human role to effect change in the universe. In other words, in contrast to an unlimited optimism about the human ability to know and bring about all things for the good, Christianity in general has asserted that human beings have a positive but limited role to play; we are not God.

Several traditional theological doctrines within Christianity come to bear upon the question of what constitutes responsible intervention in nature. First is the paradoxical assertion that human beings are both free and finite. Christian thinkers across the centuries have struggled to hold these two realities in tandem; yet, by necessity, theologians end up emphasizing one or the other of them in their efforts to make sense of the human situation. Still, even among those theologians in whose thought freedom plays a central role, it can never be severed from the fact of human finitude. For instance, in Karl Rahner's words, human freedom is always "co-determined" by our "categorical" existence (i.e., our historical existence in space and time). Thus freedom never exists in isolation, nor may it be considered unlimited; rather, it is always a response to some necessity or condition posed in time.[19]

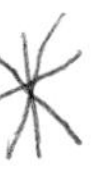

Others, delimiting the place of human freedom more sharply, have emphasized that human nature and dignity must be recognized to include not just human freedom, but also human embodiment and historical existence. Gilbert Meilaender, for instance, writes, "In our freedom we can . . . soar far above our finite condition, forgetting that there may be more ways to violate our humanity than by limiting that freedom"; and again, "To have a life is to be *terra animata,* a living body whose natural history has a trajectory."[20] Human freedom is not denied here; rather, it is contextualized by a lived, bodily existence that defines, in part, what it means to be human in the first place.

Such differing views of the role and proper use of human freedom in turn lead to two competing paradigms of how humans should intervene in nature: *stewardship* and *co-creation.* There is, of course, no neat division between these two; both draw upon biblical imagery in an effort to describe the responsibility that human beings have in relation to God's creation. Yet there is a difference in emphasis between the two that reaches directly to the heart of many questions posed by genetic manipulation.

Stewardship, a concept long used to depict the human role granted by God in the creation of the universe, places the accent on the createdness of human beings; we too are a part of God's creation, and so we are under divinely set limits on what we can and should do. God's natural order is primary. Humans are God's representatives on earth, and we are charged to live in harmony with and to care for all of creation, including human life, but this charge includes having the humility to recognize limits to our creative powers. Practicing good stewardship does not mean, however, that human beings are to refrain from exercising their creative gifts altogether. Embracing a Christian model of stewardship, Joseph D. Cassidy and Edmund D. Pellegrino maintain that there are "possibilities for human good inherent in creation," and it is the role of stewards to discern and cultivate those possibilities as best they can.[21] Accordingly, human beings are accountable to God for making use of their creative gifts as well as for the ways in which they do so.

Most accounts of co-creation, on the other hand, go a step further in their emphasis on the creative power of human beings. Here, the power to create is itself the core of the dominion that God grants to human beings. Hence, created by God, human beings are active participants in the ongoing process of creation by exercising their ability to shape, direct, even redesign nature and the process of evolution. In this way, they cooperate in creation. This is not to imply that human beings are the equivalent of God; rather, human creation *mirrors,* and thus is secondary to, divine creation. Hence, to be a co-creator lies at the very heart of what it means to be created in God's image. Moreover, God's intentions are understood to transcend what we ordinarily think of as nature so as to include active and free participation by human beings. Hence, right human action both affirms and transforms nature.

Although stewardship surely has been the predominant way that Christians have made sense of the biblical imperative of human dominion, seeds of the idea of co-creation can be found in, for example, the writings of Karl Rahner. Rahner never used the term "co-creator," but he did advocate a form of human freedom whose nature and task is essentially human self-determination. In a pair of essays, which in many ways stand in tension with one another, Rahner maintained that the human person is essentially self-creating and open to the future, and that technological self-manipulation allows us to manifest our essential freedom in the form of concrete and active neighbor-love. Yet he also argued for a certain Christian "cool-headedness" toward these technologies, and he opposed the anxious and untempered desire to plan ourselves.[22] Although there is no easy way to reconcile and integrate these two emphases, we can speculate that Rahner's overall aim was to hold the creature/co-creator poles of human nature in tension, highlighting the danger that genetic manipulation may in fact pose to human freedom and well-being. In this way Rahner represents a modified position that preserves a strong view of human freedom to intervene in nature and yet recognizes that there are limits, set by human finitude, to what may be considered good or proper forms of such intervention.

Another theological doctrine that bears upon the question of "designer" children is the place of sin in Christian theology. One could describe a spectrum of views as to the weight assigned to human sinfulness in any evaluation of genetic manipulation. In this regard, theologian James Walter contrasts two views of the Fall: (1) the view that all aspects of the human person are deeply affected by sinfulness, leading to a complete distrust of humanity's ability to make good and wise use of genetic intervention; and (2) an overly optimistic view of genetic intervention that almost entirely forgets about the effects of the Fall. In between these two extremes Walter describes a middle position (which he aligns with a moderately optimistic Roman Catholic approach): the belief that, though fallen, humanity remains essentially good and can know and do the moral good with the grace of God. According to this last view, gene therapy (even germ-line gene therapy) is not *necessarily* in violation of God's sovereignty over creation or contrary to divine purposes.[23]

At the risk of gross oversimplification, we might say that proponents of a stewardship model of human intervention generally maintain a weightier view of human sinfulness than do those who advocate a co-creationist position. The former tend to emphasize the dangers of egoism, pride, irresponsible exercise of power, and self-deception. Of course, many advocates of a more strongly co-creationist approach also highlight the human propensity to sin. In general, however, they also tend to focus more optimistically on the human ability, with the grace of God, to know and do the good, and thus to contribute positively (including by means of genetic manipulation) to an as-yet-undetermined future.[24]

A final category of Christian theology that bears upon the arguments for and against responsible intervention in nature is that of embodiment. Many contemporary Christian ethicists, responding to a traditional dualism between body and spirit, emphasize that an adequate notion of personhood must include the integral role of the human body. Whatever else the implications are of maintaining the value of the body as intrinsic to human personhood, it seems clear that human embodiment demands that we take genetic manipulation, with both its danger and its promise, seriously. Genetic manipulation is not trivial. When we intervene in the human genome, we are doing more than tinkering with the chemistry of an object; we are taking steps that may have profound effects on human personhood itself. Surely a person is more than his or her genome, but also most certainly not less. Hence, even though honoring embodiment does not dictate how we evaluate gene alteration, it does caution us against jumping into the waters of genetic manipulation too quickly and eagerly.

Arguments for Intervention

The wide variety of interpretations of the foregoing theological doctrines begins to indicate significant diversity among Christian thinkers about what constitutes responsible intervention in nature. Even among those who may be classified as "prointerventionist," it is difficult to generalize about how or why such intervention may be called for. Yet a few key arguments stand out, arguments that bear most directly on the degree to which we should allow ourselves to "shape" our offspring.

First, although individuals tend to approach the question of genetic manipulation somewhat differently, those who might qualify as prointerventionist share a basically positive stance toward the technology and a strong desire to put it to use in the service of divine purpose. At one extreme stands Protestant theologian Joseph Fletcher's early support for nearly all forms of technological control over the human condition, believing as he did that "to be civilized is to be artificial." Fletcher saw the capability for various forms of genetic engineering as basically a moral advance and advocated human control over the natural world, holding that "control as such is good, not evil, and the more the better." To be human, according to Fletcher, is to be "a maker and a selector and a designer, and the more rationally contrived and deliberate anything is, the more human it is."[25] Here, human freedom and rationality, and the ability to exercise responsible agency, are unabashedly seen as the hallmarks of what it means to be human, what sets them apart from the animals and makes them *moral* beings. Drawing on these beliefs, Fletcher enthusiastically supported most of the various sorts of reproductive and genetic technologies that he could envision at the time he wrote.

Of course, not all prointerventionist authors are as uncautiously supportive of the wide variety of reproductive and genetic technologies as Fletcher was. Lutheran theologian Ted Peters, for instance, is wary of how such technologies might go awry in the hands of sinful human beings. He cautions about the desire to design a "superior" child, and the associated potential for a loss of human dignity and psychological harm to children who are led to think of themselves as "damaged goods." Nevertheless, Peters tends to place his emphasis more on the hope and courage required of us if we are to maintain a future orientation and envision a better world. Our ethics, he maintains, should be based on our vision of the promised kingdom of God; thus our posture should be "future oriented, transformatory, active, creative, expectant, and hopeful."[26]

Underneath this shared optimistic assessment of genetic technologies lies the desire to promote human well-being as a form of loving one's neighbor. Both Fletcher and Peters place an emphasis on human welfare, and both likewise see genetic manipulation as potentially conducive to human flourishing, thus comprising our moral duty. Whereas Fletcher advocated "practical compassion" as a concrete goal of genetic manipulation, Peters argues for "beneficence" as a way of properly living out the human role as co-creators who are themselves created in God's image.[27] Unfortunately, however, neither of these authors offers much detail about the complexities of what this "practical compassion" or "beneficence" might entail with regard to "designing" our children genetically. This lack is significant because substantial disagreement can exist about what exactly constitutes "beneficence" in the complex situations that we encounter with genetic manipulation. In other words, an action that seems beneficent at first glance may in fact threaten human well-being on deeper, less readily apparent levels.

Like Fletcher and Peters, Protestant theologian Ron Cole-Turner also generally accepts a co-creationist approach to human intervention in nature and also generally supports genetic manipulation. Yet Cole-Turner arguably does a more complete job of outlining the implications of neighbor-love with respect to technologies that allow us to shape our children. For instance, he highlights Jesus' actions of healing the sick and feeding the hungry as clues about what it would mean to act redemptively vis-à-vis genetic manipulation. More than the others, he examines various dimensions of the effect that genetic manipulation could have on creaturely well-being, although his analysis is focused more on genetic screening than on the effects of genetic manipulation per se.[28]

In their common call to further God's intentions, none of these authors puts much stock into reading those intentions from nature. Fletcher argued vehemently that the artificial has been wrongly maligned by those eager to assert that nature automatically reflects what is good. The natural is not intrinsically superior to the artificial, he holds, and "to object that something is artificial only condemns it in the eyes of subrational nature lovers or natural-law mystics."[29] Nature very often brings with it misfortune, in Fletcher's view, and compassion calls us to resist such misfortune, not merely to accept it because it is "natural." Peters, with his future orientation, echoes this mistrust of deriving ethics from nature; he argues that our ethics must be "proleptic," taking its norms not from biology or nature, but rather from a heavenly vision of God's eschatological future — that is, of what life on earth *could be* if we allowed it to be influenced by a vision of the life to come.[30] Cole-Turner likewise deemphasizes nature as a source of value, viewing nature itself as fundamentally disordered. He also turns elsewhere — in this case, to Jesus' actions — to discover the norms by which we should measure our efforts.

Of course, the debate concerning the role of nature as a source for Christian ethics has a long and complex history, which I have no intention of rehearsing here. Yet it is important to note that a significant strand of Christian ethics makes a far more positive assessment of the role of nature than any of these authors do. We need not take an overly physicalist approach in order yet to maintain that careful, reasonable reflection on what appears to be "natural" and universal in human experience *can* yield significant insight into the nature of reality, thus pointing the way toward ethical norms. God's intentions need not be so cleanly divorced from what we perceive as "natural" in our world. Indeed, the final chapter of this book will seek to portray a vision of God's intentions for humanity — that is, a picture of human well-being — wherein the "natural" plays a significant role.

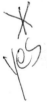

Finally, it is useful to point out that among these authors, Fletcher stands out for how little concerned he was about the phenomenon of human sinfulness. It is not that Fletcher believed that sin is absent from human action; rather, he was optimistic (perhaps overly so) that genetic manipulation can be put to use free of sin's effects. He would likely be more apt to criticize (as sinful) the tendency to draw back from genetic manipulation than the tendency to misuse it. Yet without serious discussion of the effects of human sinfulness, including the ways in which humans have erred in past usage of reproductive and genetic controls, Fletcher's uniformly optimistic evaluation of these controls very often rings hollow indeed. Peters and Cole-Turner, for their part, do not ignore human sinfulness, but they too are relatively optimistic (though not so optimistic as Fletcher) that genetic manipulation can be used well, if cautiously, by human beings in God's service.

We do better to take more seriously the dangers that human sinfulness poses vis-à-vis genetic manipulation. The history of eugenics and the tendency toward perfectionism outlined in this book certainly should give us pause before plunging ahead with an unabashedly high degree of optimism. On the one hand, greater control over the quality of human life along with an attendant reduction in human suffering certainly presents an attractive prospect; on the other hand, quality of life is a slippery concept, and, as we will see, it could be affected by genetic manipulation in ways wholly unexpected. This is particularly true as we gaze further and further into the future; the consequences of genetic manipulation are not solidly within our control. Indeed, humans may be simply unable to wield the degree of control hoped for by some.

Moreover, human sinfulness and imperfection mean that even well-intentioned efforts to improve quality of life can go awry as they are filtered through the shortcomings of finite human beings and communities. For instance, who will be exercising control over these technologies? What sort of agenda, acknowledged or unacknowledged, might they possess? How might unexamined and malicious social biases creep into the "controls" that we institute? As Maura Ryan points out, "Genetic technologies can be powerful tools for addressing human suffering. But, if in the course of attempting to eliminate genetic disease we give blessing to a 'survival of the fittest' or a 'genetic perfection' social ethic, we will have bought advancements in health at a great human cost."[31] As is evidenced by history, human sinfulness can pollute even the best of intentions.

In spite of these shortcomings, the prointerventionist accounts helpfully capture an open-ended and courageous spirit that is continuous with the hopefulness marking Christian faith. In Christian theology sin and evil never have the last word; rather, faith in the Christian God calls us to approach new situations with a spirit of hopeful expectation, even if also, at times, with caution. The theologies described above remind us that our God is, fundamentally, the God of hope and not despair, the God who empowers us to help create a better world.

Arguments for Nonintervention

The optimism of the foregoing approach is, of course, not the only way Christians have approached genetic intervention. Indeed, it is arguable that the general tenor of Christian response has been far more tempered and even pessimistic. A few influential thinkers have argued forcefully against various forms of genetic manipulation, maintaining that human intervention into nature's processes should be much more restrained than the prointerventionists allow, and their arguments have much in common.

To begin with, arguments for nonintervention tend to issue a common call to respect the dictates of nature and/or bodily existence as we evaluate the proper limits of our technological interventions. Freedom is upheld, but not nearly so strongly as in the case of prointerventionists; here, free choice is sharply limited by the contours of bodily nature and finitude. Protestant theologian Paul Ramsey, for instance, stressed that freedom is insufficient to describe the human person and is an inadequate basis, on its own, to guide our ethical choices; the *humanum* includes also our sexual, bodily nature, and the biological is not simply to be dominated and controlled, but rather respected.[32] Another Protestant theologian, Gilbert Meilaender, picks up the theme, emphasizing that human freedom is tempered by an embodiment that importantly defines who we are and what our possibilities are. Intervention in nature may be appropriate, "for such self-transcendence is an expression of the freedom that is essential to being human"; yet "neither should we assume . . . that freedom is the sole truth about our nature." Such intervention, in Meilaender's view, must be thoughtful and limited because "any particular step may be the one that we should not take, the one that will destroy something as essential to our humanity as freedom is."[33] Clearly, both of these authors represent a sharp break with the relatively wide scope of freedom advocated by strongly liberal thought.

These authors are also marked by a common call to hold together the unitive and procreative dimensions of sexual love. Ramsey believed that procreation is designed to take place as an extension of the love between a husband and a wife, and in that union he saw "a trace of the original mystery by which God created the world because of His love."[34] According to this understanding of the nature of parenthood, which Ramsey called "a basic form of humanity," it is wrong to separate these two goods; that is, it is wrong to view procreation as a matter for technical control and its unitive purpose as entirely subject to our free choice. Thus, to treat procreation as purely a matter for technical control, separate from personal love and sexual relations, is to distort its intrinsic meaning and ultimately will depersonalize human life together. This concern is echoed by theologian Oliver O'Donovan, who fears the day when sexual activity might be understood as being entirely subject to the human will, thus breaking the connection between procreation and sexual intercourse, and wrongly turning a natural process into a purely technological undertaking. When we do this, he argues, we run the risk that children become our *projects,* rather than the mysterious possibilities that spring from our love.

The implications of this approach are most obvious in the case of reproductive technologies such as artificial insemination by donor or in vitro fertilization. Yet even genetic manipulation is affected insofar as these technologies transform procreation from a natural "by-product" of sexual love into a detailed technological process subject to the dictates of human will. Noninterventionists tend to reject or sharply restrict genetic manipulations that encourage or allow us to disregard nature's limits and to view ourselves as proper designers of human life. In their view, these would dangerously depersonalize procreation and very likely harm the children who result.

Again, then, the question arises: Do these technologies of genetic manipulation depersonalize procreation? It is important to note that these noninterventionist theologians at times make relatively arbitrary distinctions about what constitutes unacceptable human control. Maura Ryan, for instance, criticizes Ramsey's tendency to disparage medically assisted reproduction using (negatively) the rhetoric of "mastery"; this merely begs the ethical question, she holds, for he lacks a good account of why and exactly how proposed interventions slip over the line of acceptability.[35] Ramsey himself embraced what he termed "genetic surgery," if it could be made safe: microsurgery to eliminate genetic defects in parents before they can be passed on through reproduction. Yet he also clearly opposed any impulse toward viewing procreation as a process of manufacture, engineering, or "genetic tailoring"; this would be to "play God" and would help drive a dangerous wedge between the biological and the "personal" aspects of human procreation.

Another problem with this approach lies in its perhaps overly heavy emphasis on the biological or physical dimensions of human existence. Indeed, here, one of its greatest strengths, the attention to human embodiedness, sometimes can become a weakness. An overemphasis on the physical aspects of human procreation can result in an unwillingness to tamper with it at all, effectively eliminating the possibilities for furthering human welfare that many forms of gene therapy offer. Ramsey and Meilaender, at least, do not make this error, for they recognize that human freedom can be a powerful ally of neighbor-love if used wisely; still, it can be argued that their analyses at times underplay this role of human freedom too greatly.

Perhaps the most important point to be taken away from the non-interventionist stances described here is that we should not move hastily toward embracing techniques of genetic control. Before seeking mastery over the human genome, we should step back and look for the good that *is:* the good of creation, of what is natural and given. Meilaender puts the point best, arguing that what we need is not total control over our offspring, but rather a renewed respect for the mystery of personhood as it unfolds in a child:

> To conceive, bear, give birth to, and rear a child ought to be an affirmation and a recognition: affirmation of the good of life that we ourselves were given; recognition that this life bears its own creative power to which we should be faithful.... That a new human being should come into existence is not ultimately our doing. Within this life we can exercise a modest degree of control, but if we seek to do more than that we have fundamentally altered the nature of what we are doing — and of the beings to whom we give rise.[36]

Here, it seems that the nature of parenthood and the good of children are at stake. Although there are times that intervening in, and thus controlling, nature may be called for, we must realize that we risk losing something important when we try to control *everything* about procreation. Moreover, when we look for the good in creation, we should look deeply, for sometimes it is difficult to see at first glance the good that in fact exists in creation, particularly when that creation is marked by pain and suffering. Christian faith does not call us to stand still, but it does call us to move cautiously, to use our freedom wisely, and to pause before we too quickly deny the good of God's created order.

Negotiating the Rift

How are we to negotiate such fundamentally different approaches to appropriate human intervention in nature, particularly in the realm of genetic manipulation of children? Although the differences are vast among the aforementioned approaches, we can seek to unite their strengths and, in so doing, try to identify a Christian posture of limited, responsible intervention in nature.

From those who are relatively more sympathetic to genetic intervention, we learn the importance in Christian thought of hopefulness, and thus of optimism toward our possibilities as partners in God's creative processes. Christian faith, it seems, urges that our actions be based not on fear, but rather on a positive, hopeful, and empowered posture toward the possibilities that God sets before us. We also are reminded of the tremendous possibilities for acting out neighbor-love that genetic technologies offer us: the chance to dramatically reduce human suffering. Finally, we should be cautioned against too quickly or easily resigning ourselves to what seems to be the "God-given" dictates of nature, realizing instead that God's intentions sometimes transcend physical or biological reality.

On the other hand, those who take a more cautious or conservative posture toward genetic intervention remind us that we must yet pay attention to what nature has to teach us. A misguided attempt utterly to deny nature's limits contradicts our embodied, historical existence. If we move too quickly toward a constant focus on changing and manipulating nature to our advantage, we will miss much of the beauty and value of life that is bound up with our limited, bodily existence, and sometimes even bound up with our misfortune. We will be more likely to miss, for instance, the spiritual significance of having children, in the rush to have a particular *kind* of child. We will be more likely to miss the lessons that the less-than-perfect (e.g., persons with retardation) have to teach us. We will be more likely to miss out on the virtue and satisfaction that follow when we accept, learn to live with, and learn *from* our children's faults.

The foregoing theological positions also remind us, in their separate ways, to beware of human sinfulness. In the face of genetic technologies, sin could take the form of complacency and a fearful rejection of change, on the one hand, or of hubris, an overdeveloped sense of control, and the will to power, on the other. Again, our shameful history of eugenic control and the contemporary perfectionist attitudes toward children should caution us about some of the potentially sinful abuses of technologies of genetic manipulation. We need a more prominent red flag here than many co-creationists are apt to raise. Still, sin and evil do not have the last word, and our attentiveness toward their insidious danger should not keep us from recognizing when we are called to exercise our creative powers and *act*.

Taken together, these lessons point toward a posture whereby we seek a reflective balance between learning from nature and seeking to change nature, a balance similar to the creature/co-creator tension that we found in the writings of Rahner, for instance. Without moving rashly toward change, and toward our visions of the "perfect" child, we must yet seek to discern when change is called for. This means that we must value and honor, not fear, our freedom, but we must be prepared at times to say no to certain exercises of freedom that would be inconsistent with our best discernment of the divine intent for creation. Throughout, we must remain aware of the ways that we are prone, individually and societally, to act in contradiction to God's intention.

As we begin to do this, it is my contention that genetic intervention should be guided, in large part, by the best interests of the children who would be "designed." This involves looking deeply and carefully at the best interests of such children, at how they will be affected not only physically, but also psychologically and socially. Moreover, it means that we must evaluate the effect that genetic manipulation would have on society's (and families') attitudes toward these children, and toward parenthood in general. It seems possible that some interventions would indeed alter how we as a society and as individuals understand parenthood, while others would not do so, or would do so less, or would do so while simultaneously bringing about great benefit to a child. Finally, the sorts of genetic manipulation that we accept should serve the value of neighbor-love, not parental fearfulness, as we seek to "better" the lives of our children.

These considerations will be more fully fleshed out in the next chapter of this book, where I will more directly address the concept of human flourishing on individual and social levels. Before turning to that project, however, there is one final Christian theme to be examined, a theme that is an integral part of human flourishing and bears directly on the issue of genetic manipulation: the Christian affirmation of the common good.

The Common Good and Genetic Manipulation

In a persuasive essay on the "twinning" of human embryos, Roman Catholic moral theologian Richard McCormick critiques the liberal individualist posture embraced by John Robertson and implicitly adopted by much of modern Western society, a posture that he interprets to hold that an individual's (or a couple's) autonomous desire to overcome infertility trumps all other considerations. McCormick maintains, "Once our culture views human persons as isolated and autonomous agents — as it does — then nearly anything becomes thinkable."[37] McCormick's central point here is that we need to examine the social context and impact of any proposed intervention, for at stake is not only the possible good or harm done to the individual who chooses to make use of the technology, but also the positive or negative consequences for the common good. Moreover, it does not make sense for us to think of persons in isolation from this common good, since that is simply not how real persons exist.

The common good is, in fact, a persistent theme within Christianity. Over and over again, from the apostle Paul's exhortations to think of ourselves as one "body" (of Christ) to the emphasis by various later theologians, most prominently in the Roman Catholic tradition, on the common good and its place in the social order, Christianity as a whole does not support radical individualism. Considering and supporting the good of the larger community or society is a prominent feature of how Christians are to approach any given issue.

In the case of the genetic shaping of offspring, this means that the individual rights and well-being of would-be parents and children must not be radically disassociated from the creation and preservation of a just social order. What exactly this means will, of course, depend on the existing contours of our political and social life together. At a bare minimum, there are three dimensions of the contemporary U.S. social order to attend to in regard to genetic technologies: (1) the distribution of scarce healthcare dollars toward these technologies; (2) the distribution of the technologies themselves; and, perhaps most troubling, (3) certain harmful social inequalities that genetic manipulation might aggravate. I will briefly consider each in turn.

The Use of Scarce Resources for Genetic Manipulation

The financial troubles of the U.S. healthcare system in recent years are, by now, old news. As stated in previous chapters, over forty-one million people in the United States are uninsured, and many more lack full access to the healthcare system. Hence, inadequate healthcare is a hallmark of the early twenty-first-century United States. Many people lack even the most basic health services, services that would ward off later, more expensive measures. These basic services include prenatal and well-baby care, and disease prevention and health promotion. Needless to say, addressing this calamity has been a major topic of public policy discussion for the past decade.

In the midst of this healthcare turmoil, it must be asked whether genetic manipulation of offspring deserves to be prioritized financially. Although it is true that genetic diseases collectively do account for a great deal of human suffering, most individual genetic diseases are fairly rare, relative to nongenetic diseases. Moreover, as research advances, no doubt a good deal of effort will be poured into the lucrative markets associated with sex selection and genetic enhancement. Funding such seemingly trivial choices as the birth order of boys and girls, or the esoteric pursuit of enhanced memory capabilities in a child, seems irresponsible in a society in which millions of people cannot even afford to feed their children properly.

For Christians, such choices may not be simply irresponsible; they may, in fact, contradict the will of God. Many Christians agree that God "takes the side of," or makes a "preferential option" for, the poor. Hence, every policy decision must be evaluated from the standpoint of social justice. Along these lines, Allen Verhey criticizes the allocation of resources to the Human Genome Project, asking,

> When cities are crumbling, when schools are deteriorating, when we complain about not having sufficient resources to help the poor or the homeless, when we do not have the resources to provide care for all the sick, is this a just and fair use of our society's resources? Is it an allocation of social resources that can claim to imitate God's care and concern for the poor?[38]

Here, Verhey questions the overall distribution of a budget favoring high-technology "fixes" that seem to do little concretely to address the struggles of poor persons and communities. Moreover, even within a fixed budget for healthcare, a relatively expensive focus on identifying the genetic mutations associated with various human characteristics may preclude less exotic efforts at ensuring that basic healthcare needs are met for low-income or otherwise disenfranchised people. In this way, genetic manipulation could function to reinforce their social marginalization.

In light of this view on genetic manipulation, Christian faith calls us to make careful choices about precisely which genetic interventions are warranted expenditures of our healthcare dollars. If distinctions are indeed to be made, preventing genetic diseases that cause immense or widespread suffering will be more justifiable than seeking to enhance memory, or to dictate eye or skin color, or even to preselect gender. Furthermore, expenditures on genetic technologies as a whole should not eclipse the urgent need to address poverty and poverty-related illness and misfortune in our society, the vast majority of which is completely unrelated to genetic disease.

The Distribution of Genetic Technologies

Even if we decide that scarce healthcare dollars should be allocated toward technologies of genetic manipulation, the question remains as to how justly those technologies themselves are distributed. In other words, which kinds of genetic manipulations will receive attention? Who will share in the benefits of these technologies if and when they ultimately are perfected for use? Are they the same persons and communities who have borne the burdens and the risks?

In the liberal market society of the United States it is undeniable that market considerations have driven genetic research. Hence, as Lisa Sowle Cahill points out, there has been no significant genetic research on malaria, since Africa, where the disease is most prevalent, is not a lucrative market. Similarly, genetic research to combat muscular dystrophy has been sought out by some who wish to offer it to healthy U.S. athletes so that they might grow larger muscles; and researchers in gene therapy have been approached by doctors who wish to offer their patients the chance genetically to alter their racial appearance.[39] In these cases, technologies of genetic manipulation are pursued for their financial promise, with the result that markets, not justice, are likely to drive exactly which technologies are developed.

From the standpoint of marginalized communities, this is, for the most part, not good news. Though many poor people suffer from genetic diseases, there is no guarantee that the research done will focus on those diseases at all; indeed, it may well favor genetic enhancement for cosmetic or other purposes, since that is where much of the money is to be had. Moreover, will the poor ultimately have access to these techniques of genetic manipulation, techniques for which their tax dollars helped pay? Given the radical disparity of healthcare distribution under our current system, there is little reason to believe that genetic manipulation will be widely available to anyone but the relatively rich, and certainly not to those without reasonably good access to health insurance.

Christian faith calls us to challenge this unequal distribution of the benefits of genetic technology. If we as a society elect to continue to sustain the research backing genetic manipulation, then we must ensure that all members of society have access to its benefits, or at least those benefits that support a basic quality of life. What exactly this might include will be addressed in the final chapter of this book. Here it is sufficient to note that Christianity calls us to view the distribution of genetic technologies, like all social policies, with the eyes of the most socially vulnerable among us.

Potential Aggravation of Harmful Social Inequalities

The final, and most troubling, category of concerns falling under the general consideration of the common good has to do with existent social inequalities that techniques of genetic manipulation might aggravate. Many have recognized the danger; in fact, Pope John Paul II, in his address to the World Medical Association in 1983, urged that we avoid any manipulations that tend to create groups of different people at the risk of provoking fresh marginalization in society. Karl Rahner was even more alarmed about possible new social tensions; he cautioned that genetic manipulation could lead to two new "races" in humankind: "superbred" humans and ordinary, unselected ones.[40] Finally, a 1997 *Washington Post* article put the matter bluntly: "Might [cosmetic gene therapy] lead to a society of DNA haves and have-nots, and the creation of a new underclass of people unable to keep up with the genetically fortified Joneses?"[41] At stake in all these cases is a fundamental commitment that Christian tradition makes to oppose gross social disparities, which undermine the equal dignity of all human beings.

Whether or not an entire social class of superbred human beings is a likely possibility, it does seem probable that widespread use of genetic technologies to "design" children could reinforce existing economic and social divisions. Again, those most likely to make use of such technologies are those with sufficient economic resources to gain access to them. Michael Langan, former vice president of the National Organization for Rare Disorders, has expressed his fear that genetic manipulation will lead to a society in which those who cannot afford the technology are ostracized for their imperfections:

> There will be many wealthy people willing and eager to pay the price of making their child taller and more beautiful. . . . Eventually there will be discrimination against those who look "different" because their genes were not altered. The absence of ethical restraints means crooked noses and teeth, or acne, or baldness, will become the mark of Cain in a century from now.[42]

Beyond the economic question, there is the problem that racial, gender, and other forms of social discrimination still pose in contemporary Western society; genetic manipulation represents yet another tool, and a potent one, by which such harmful social patterns can gain an even stronger foothold. Ethicist Eric Juengst states the danger: "Self-improvement and wanting the best for your children is acceptable and encouraged in this culture. . . . But would I be complicitous with some unfair cultural values if I choose to change my skin color to one that offers the best chances of societal acceptance?"[43]

Indeed, to the degree that such possibilities for change are embraced by a large segment of the population, increased social discrimination seems a likely outcome. This is especially troubling in light of the history of eugenics in this country and the contemporary impetus toward perfectionism described in the second chapter of this book. As Jewish ethicist Laurie Zoloth-Dorfman has pointed out, in this country visible differences have historically been used as a signifier not just of *difference,* but also of *exclusion,* with demonstrable negative health effects on those who are excluded.[44] Although others have rightly argued that prejudice and discrimination thrive even without genetic manipulation, genetic technologies could in fact powerfully reinforce a problem that we as a society would do better to fight against.

The issue of increased discrimination resulting from genetic manipulation has been of particular concern to the disabled-rights community. A reasonable fear exists that the advent of genetic manipulation will translate into an increasingly hostile environment for persons with physical or mental disabilities. In other words, as the possibility for using genetic manipulation to prevent disability becomes more realistic, there exists a corresponding danger that social tolerance for the needs of the disabled themselves will wane, as will public willingness to invest in changes that would make our social order more open and accessible to those with disabilities.

Along these lines, Stanley Hauerwas points out that modern medicine, in its quest to reduce suffering, can instead become the means by which we unjustly eliminate, in the name of humanity, those who suffer. He argues that a great deal of the suffering of persons with retardation is actually due to the fact that they live in a hostile world; thus the task should be to change the nature of the world, not to eliminate the persons themselves. Avoiding this truth is a matter of profound self-deception, in Hauerwas' view. He writes, "Too often the suffering we wish to spare [persons with retardation] is the result of our unwillingness to change our lives so that those disabled might have a better life."[45] Here, genetic prevention of disability might be viewed as yet another misguided attempt to escape from the responsibility that we as a community have to make our world a more welcoming and hospitable place.

Social intolerance for those with disabilities may even appear in the form of criticism of parents who choose *not* to make use of genetic manipulation techniques. Moral theologian Eberhard Schockenhoff, for instance, expresses the fear that "one will have to justify oneself before society for the mere existence of a handicapped child, the acceptance of which one could have spared oneself and the community."[46] Indeed, if genetic manipulation allows parents to avoid disabilities in their children, no doubt there will be enormous social pressure for parents to use it; and this likely will become increasingly true as society becomes decreasingly accommodating of persons with disabilities. For instance, if publicly funded programs for persons with retardation are given less and less social support, it will seem, to everyone, an even greater burden for parents to bring into the world a child disabled in this way. The end result is hardly a society characterized by an open and welcoming attitude toward disabled persons, or a valuing of the basic equality of each human being.

In opposing these sorts of social inequalities, many contemporary Christian thinkers uphold the value of diversity as bound up with the common good. Among these is Richard McCormick, who emphasizes that human "uniqueness and diversity (sexual, racial, ethnic, and cultural) are treasured aspects of the human condition," reflecting the image of God. He argues that we must resist any diagnostic or eugenic interventions that would "bypass, downplay, or flatten these diversities and uniqueness," paradoxically at a time when elsewhere we are emphasizing them.[47] Indeed, the sordid history of racial, sexual, and cultural groups falsely imposing their particularities as universals has led to a widespread cry in "postmodern" culture asserting the value of diversity.

Others who oppose unlimited genetic intervention often point out how diversity itself acts as a sort of insurance against the unexpected, since certain traits may be called for in the future, traits for which we see no positive use today.[48] Genetic diversity is considered important to the survival of the human race because it allows us to survive and adapt to new situations. Moreover, deviations from what is considered "normal" (such as the genetic mutation responsible for sickle-cell trait) sometimes have been found to convey benefits previously unrecognized (in this case, a resistance to malaria). Along these lines, there is some evidence that the genetic mutation responsible for cystic fibrosis also offers some protection against typhoid fever.[49] Hence, to scoff at or downplay the value of human diversity is to fail to recognize the ways in which we are dependent on diversity for our well-being.

It is important, however, to recognize that diversity itself is not an unlimited value. A commitment to oppose harmful social inequalities or uphold human diversity does not mean that we must accept all forms of variation in human existence. Roger Shinn, for instance, points out that "diversifying can come at too great a cost," and that "there are diseases that nobody would deliberately perpetuate for the sake of human diversity" or because they might have some unknown survival value for descendants in a transformed environment.[50] Rather, we must seek to discern *when* genetic manipulation will be likely to create or exacerbate harmful inequalities or threaten the beauty of human diversity.

Furthermore, we must weigh the benefits of different forms of genetic manipulation (e.g., the reduction of suffering) against the danger that it will reduce human and genetic diversity. These are not easy distinctions to make, but they are necessary if we are serious about protecting and promoting not simply individual free choice or well-being, but also the goods wrapped up in our common life.

Implications for the Shaping of Children

The foregoing considerations point us toward a vision of personal and social relationships profoundly different from a purely liberal individualist approach. According to Christian wisdom, there is more to human procreation than the exercise of our rational wills, and there exist certain appropriate limits to our free choice in the realm of procreation. In fact, it is God's intentions, however difficult they may be to discern, that begin to set the parameters for how we may intervene in human genetic processes.

To begin with, Christianity discerns that God does not intend for us to seek absolute control over a child. According to Christianity, a child is not properly understood as the object of ownership or rational design, or as existing primarily to meet the needs of his or her parents. Rather, children, like all human beings, are created in the image of God; they possess independent value and dignity, and indeed they are precious in God's sight. Hence, they are gifted into our care as part of a divinely granted vocation. So it is that children above all merit our awe, respect, and unconditional love, long before we engage in any efforts to alter who they are, genetically or otherwise.

Moreover, as part of that vocation, we are called to discern as best we can where exactly the best interests of children lie vis-à-vis any given form of genetic manipulation, for most Christians agree that the promotion of human well-being is a crucial part of God's intention for creation. Such discernment will include evaluating not only the effects of genetic manipulation on the immediate well-being of children, but also the effects that such technologies will have on the broader relationships that those children hold, including relationships to parents and to the wider society. If the widespread availability of genetic manipulation means that many parents will begin to understand parenthood itself less as the acceptance of a calling and more as a sort of shopping expedition, then Christian faith calls us to challenge that understanding.

Finally, Christianity understands the common good to be an integral part of God's intention for the world, and it challenges any use of genetic manipulation that threatens that common good by deepening social or economic stratification or by flattening out the wondrous diversity that characterizes the human community. Because individuals, including both children and their parents, cannot be isolated from the larger societies of which they are a part, it is meaningless to promote their best interests apart from the broader contours of social well-being. Moreover, according to Christian faith, we should have particular concern for the effect of genetic manipulation on marginalized communities, and we must take steps to insure that the risks and benefits associated with genetic technologies are justly distributed.

If Christianity provides us reasons to hesitate before plunging into the use of genetic manipulation, however, it also provides us with excellent reasons not to shun it altogether. Christianity is not a religion of fear or complacency. It is, rather, a religion that calls us to act on our beliefs, a faith that empowers us to exercise our abilities in order to help reduce human suffering and create a world more in line with divine intent. Some forms of genetic manipulation hold immense promise to relieve or prevent profound forms of human suffering, and we must not flee from this promise prematurely. Again, the co-creationists remind us that the Christian God calls for a spirit of hope, not despair, and genetic technologies offer us new possibilities for acting on that hope. Although we must recognize creaturely limits to the exercise of our freedom, we still have a certain responsibility as partners in the creative process.

When we turn more directly to the various sorts of genetic manipulation, these guidelines seem to affirm that greater caution is called for as we move further along the continuum from healing to enhancement.

That is, the further removed we are from preventing the obvious suffering of people, the more questionable our interventions will be. Quite obviously, the well-being of a child with severe cystic fibrosis is compromised in a way that the well-being of a child with average memory or intelligence most often is not. Hence, it is possible that the needs of the child with cystic fibrosis merit that we risk the pitfalls of genetic intervention, while the "needs" of more ordinary children do not merit such risk. The Christian story reminds us that Jesus acted to *heal*, not to give people a "leg up" over others in the world.

Sex preselection poses more complications. Many of the concerns raised in previous chapters about sex preselection would be affirmed by a Christian concern to support human dignity and well-being and to foster the common good. In addition, there is nothing normatively questionable, from a Christian perspective, about the existence of both males and females, and both are rightly affirmed as reflecting the image of God. Hence, there would seem to be no good reason to intervene genetically for the sole purpose of preselecting offspring sex. On the other hand, there are cases where immense human suffering and even death is tied to, or occasioned by, the mere fact of being either male or female. This is especially true with sex-linked genetic disease, where a Christian mandate to relieve suffering may lead us to affirm sex preselection. Sex-linked human suffering also exists, of course, in many developing countries, where girl children are at much higher risk of infanticide or malnutrition. The argument sometimes is made that the relief of human suffering *here* dictates that sex preselection be allowed in order to reduce the incidence of this sort of suffering. This possibility will be explored further in the final chapter of this book, as I explicate the meaning of human flourishing in the context of different forms of genetic manipulation, including sex preselection.

In these ways, the aforementioned guidelines begin to inform us about how to make distinctions between various sorts of genetic manipulation. Yet before we can truly make an adequate evaluation, we need more than general affirmations of the dignity and value of children, or of human well-being, or of the value of social diversity. We need to specify a more concrete and detailed picture of human flourishing, one that helps us to determine when the best interests of children are being honored, or when the values that characterize human welfare within families are being upheld. Moreover, a *feminist* Christian approach will also take into consideration the concerns for women's well-being articulated in chapter 3. Let us therefore turn squarely to explicating such a picture and applying it to various sorts of genetic manipulation.

Notes

1. Georgia Harkness, *John Calvin: The Man and His Ethics* (New York: Abingdon, 1931), 145.

2. John Robertson, *Children of Choice: Freedom and the New Reproductive Technologies* (Princeton, N. J.: Princeton University Press, 1994), 5.

3. It is somewhat misleading to speak of "the Christian tradition" as if it presents a monolithic view on this subject or any other. Nevertheless, it is my contention that the tradition as a whole generally supports certain themes, identified here, that are particularly relevant to the discussion at hand. Even within these themes, as will become apparent, there exists a diversity of thought among Christians. My aim here is to negotiate this diversity in order to arrive at certain normative guidelines by which to evaluate particular cases of genetic manipulation.

4. Martin Luther, "The Estate of Marriage," in *Luther's Works,* vol. 45, ed. Walther I. Brandt (Philadelphia: Fortress, 1962), 46; see also "A Sermon on the Estate of Marriage," in *Luther's Works,* vol. 44, ed. James Atkinson (Philadelphia: Fortress, 1966), 3–14.

5. Karen Lebacqz, ed., *Genetics, Ethics and Parenthood* (New York: Pilgrim Press, 1983), 18; James M. Gustafson, *Ethics from a Theocentric Perspective,* vol. 2, *Ethics and Theology* (Chicago: University of Chicago Press, 1984), 167.

6. Maura A. Ryan, "The Argument for Unlimited Procreative Liberty: A Feminist Critique," *Hastings Center Report* 20, no. 4 (1990): 10.

7. Courtney S. Campbell, "Prophecy and Policy," *Hastings Center Report* 27, no. 5 (1997): 16. Paul Ramsey refers to the "poetry" and the "surprise" of a child in his refutation of in vitro fertilization. See Paul Ramsey, "Manufacturing Our Offspring: Weighing the Risks," *Hastings Center Report* 8, no. 5 (1978): 9.

8. Gilbert Meilaender, *Bioethics: A Primer for Christians* (Grand Rapids: Eerdmans, 1996), 45.

9. Thomas A. Shannon, "Ethical Issues in Genetics," *Theological Studies* 60 (1999): 122. Although Shannon does not reject these technologies outright, he does raise a note of caution about how we make use of them.

10. Stanley Hauerwas, *Truthfulness and Tragedy: Further Investigations into Christian Ethics* (Notre Dame, Ind.: University of Notre Dame Press, 1977), 150.

11. Stanley Hauerwas, *Suffering Presence: Theological Reflections on Medicine, the Mentally Handicapped, and the Church* (Notre Dame, Ind.: University of Notre Dame Press, 1986), 215.

12. Stanley Hauerwas, *A Community of Character: Toward a Constructive Christian Social Ethic* (Notre Dame, Ind.: University of Notre Dame Press, 1981), 227.

13. Gilbert Meilaender, "Mastering our Gen(i)es: When Do We Say No?" *Christian Century,* October 3, 1990, 874–75.

14. World Council of Churches, *Manipulating Life: Ethical Issues in Genetic Engineering* (Geneva: World Council of Churches, 1982), 7.

15. Richard A. McCormick, S.J., "Blastomere Separation: Some Concerns," *Hastings Center Report* 24, no. 2 (1994): 15.

16. Oliver O'Donovan, *Begotten or Made?* (Oxford: Clarendon, 1984), 65.

17. United Church of Christ, "Pronouncement: Church and Genetic Engineering," in *Minutes of the Seventeenth General Synod* (United Church of Christ, 1989), 42; Allen Verhey, "'Playing God' and Invoking a Perspective," *Journal of Medicine and Philosophy* 20 (1995): 361.

18. Hauerwas, *Suffering Presence,* 168.

19. Karl Rahner, *Foundations of Christian Faith: An Introduction to the Idea of Christianity,* trans. William V. Dych (New York: Crossroad, 1994), 97; "The Dignity and Freedom of Man," in *Theological Investigations,* vol. 2, *Man in the Church,* trans. K.-H. Kruger (Baltimore: Helicon, 1963), 247; "Theology of Freedom," in *Theological Investigations,* vol. 6, *Concerning Vatican Council II,* trans. K.-H. Kruger and B. Kruger (New York: Seabury, 1974), 194.

20. Gilbert Meilaender, *Body, Soul, and Bioethics* (Notre Dame, Ind.: University of Notre Dame Press, 1995), 80, 56.

21. Joseph D. Cassidy and Edmund D. Pellegrino, "A Catholic Perspective on Human Gene Therapy," *International Journal of Bioethics* 4, no. 1 (1993): 12.

22. Karl Rahner, "The Experiment with Man: Theological Observations on Man's Self-Manipulation" and "The Problem of Genetic Manipulation," in *Theological Investigations,* vol. 9, *Writings of 1965–1967, I,* trans. D. Bourke (New York: Herder & Herder, 1972), 205–24 and 225–52 (respectively).

23. James J. Walter, "'Playing God' or Properly Exercising Human Responsibility? Some Theological Reflections on Human Germ-Line Therapy," *New Theology Review* 10, no. 4 (1997): 49.

24. See, for instance, Ted Peters, "'Playing God' and Germline Intervention," *Journal of Medicine and Philosophy* 20 (1995): 365–86; *For the Love of Children: Genetic Technology and the Future of the Family* (Louisville: Westminster John Knox, 1996); *Playing God? Genetic Determinism and Human Freedom* (New York: Routledge, 1997); Thomas A. Shannon, *What Are They Saying About Genetic Engineering?* (New York: Paulist Press, 1985); Ronald Cole-Turner, *The New Genesis: Theology and the Genetic Revolution* (Louisville: Westminster John Knox, 1993).

25. Joseph Fletcher, *The Ethics of Genetic Control: Ending Reproductive Roulette* (Garden City, N.Y.: Anchor Books, 1974), 15, 183; "Ethical Aspects of Genetic Controls: Designed Genetic Changes in Man," *New England Journal of Medicine* 285, no. 14 (1971): 780.

26. Peters, *For the Love of Children,* 155.

27. Fletcher, *Ethics of Genetic Control,* 159; Peters, *Playing God?* 161.

28. Ronald Cole-Turner, *The New Genesis: Theology and the Genetic Revolution* (Louisville: Westminster John Knox, 1993), 93; see also Cole-Turner, "Is Genetic Engineering

Co-Creation?" *Theology Today* 44 (October 1987): 338–49; Ronald Cole-Turner and Brent Waters, *Pastoral Genetics: Theology and Care at the Beginning of Life* (Cleveland: Pilgrim Press, 1996).

29. Fletcher, *Ethics of Genetic Control,* 15.

30. Peters, *For the Love of Children,* 182.

31. Maura A. Ryan, "Feminist Theology and the New Genetics," in *The Ethics of Genetic Engineering,* ed. Maureen Junker-Kenny and Lisa Sowle Cahill (London: SCM Press, 1998), 98.

32. Paul Ramsey, *Fabricated Man: The Ethics of Genetic Control* (New Haven: Yale University Press, 1970), 31.

33. Meilaender, "Mastering our Gen(i)es," 872.

34. Ramsey, *Fabricated Man,* 88.

35. Maura A. Ryan, "The New Reproductive Technologies: Defying God's Dominion?" *Journal of Medicine and Philosophy* 20 (1995): 423.

36. Meilaender, *Body, Soul, and Bioethics,* 84–85.

37. McCormick, "Blastomere Separation," 16.

38. Verhey, " 'Playing God,' " 361.

39. Lisa Sowle Cahill, "Genetics, Ethics and Social Policy: The State of the Question," in Junker-Kenney and Cahill, eds., *Ethics of Genetic Engineering,* xi.

40. John Paul II, "The Ethics of Genetic Manipulation," *Origins* 13, no. 23 (1983): 388; Rahner, "Problem of Genetic Manipulation," 246.

41. Rick Weiss, "Gene Enhancements' Thorny Ethical Traits," *Washington Post,* October 12, 1997, A1.

42. Quoted in ibid., A19.

43. Quoted in ibid.

44. Laurie Zoloth-Dorfman, "Mapping the Normal Human Self: The Jew and the Mark of Otherness," in *Genetics: Issues of Social Justice,* ed. Ted Peters (Cleveland: Pilgrim Press, 1998), 196.

45. Hauerwas, *Suffering Presence,* 173; see also 160, 172.

46. Eberhard Schockenhoff, "First Sheep, Then Human Beings? Theological and Ethical Reflections on the Use of Gene Technology," in Junker-Kenney and Cahill, eds., *Ethics of Genetic Engineering,* 88.

47. Richard McCormick, "Genetic Technology and Our Common Future," in *The Critical Calling: Reflections on Moral Dilemmas Since Vatican II* (Washington, D.C.: Georgetown University Press, 1989), 268–69.

48. Roger Lincoln Shinn, *The New Genetics: Challenges for Science, Faith, and Politics* (Wakefield, R.I.: Moyer Bell, 1996), 113.

49. G. B. Pier et al., "Salmonella Typhi Uses CFTR to Enter Intestinal Epithelial Cells," *Nature* 393 (1998): 79–82.

50. Shinn, *New Genetics,* 114, 134.

Chapter Five

Procreation and Human Flourishing

When all that says "it is good" has been debunked, what says "I want" remains. — C. S. Lewis[1]

According to the analysis of this book, the best insights of both feminism and Christian faith point us away from the unlimited and unconditional use of genetic manipulation. Procreative liberty surely has an important role to play in feminist moral analysis and commitments, but as we have seen, the particular type of feminism embraced here reaches beyond a myopic focus on procreative liberty to embrace and advocate a more complete picture of human well-being. Similarly, Christian faith upholds the value of human freedom, on the one hand, and medical interventions that are designed to support the health and well-being of persons, on the other; nevertheless, it raises multiple red flags when it comes to the matter of *unlimited* choice in the selection of offspring characteristics.

From these points of view, procreative liberty must not stand alone as a guiding value in human reproduction. Rather than embracing reproductive control as an unmitigated good, both feminist and Christian thought, as interpreted here, point toward the wisdom of accepting some limits on how far we human beings should attempt to shape our offspring genetically. At the same time, neither feminist nor Christian thought would be true to its own best insights if it were to do away with procreative liberty altogether, for such freedom contributes in important ways to individual and social well-being and represents one significant manifestation of human co-creativity.

The goal of the present chapter is to negotiate these tensions by offering a normative account of human flourishing with respect to procreation and parent-child relations, an account that is consistent with the best insights of the feminist and Christian visions offered in previous chapters. This account will allow us to begin to establish more clearly what are the proper limits when it comes to the choice to manipulate our offspring genetically. In the final chapter I will turn again to the concrete issues of disease prevention, memory enhancement, and sex preselection, examining each in light of the vision of human flourishing that I offer, and seeking to arrive at some provisional conclusions about the wisdom of allowing or encouraging these particular forms of genetic intervention.

Postmodernism and Human Well-Being

Articulating any normative account of human flourishing that purports to address more than a very limited group of people is a dangerous business in an age of postmodernism. A postmodernist celebration of "otherness" and difference has assailed previous efforts to articulate and advance shared moral norms, rightfully judging that these too often have promoted false "universals" and ignored the tremendous importance of human particularity and situatedness. This is a particularly incisive critique from the point of view of feminism, for feminists have long understood that the "universal" human being on which much of moral theory has been patterned has in fact been a *male* human being and thus has inadequately reflected women's experience. Even within feminism itself an anti-essentialist critique has pointed out the ways that feminist thought has wrongly generalized about "women's" experience without attending to the many and varied kinds of experiences among women. The deconstructionist insight that moral foundationalism has at times obscured the complex moral texture of human life makes it difficult to put forth any positive vision of human flourishing that spans culture, place, or time to any significant degree.

Nevertheless, neither feminist nor Christian moral theory can afford to forsake the effort. As Christina Traina points out, the thoroughgoing attack on moral realism often associated with the postmodernist critique "entails the 'loss of any fixed base from which to engage in moral assessment,' like minimal standards of justice or visions of human flourishing"; Margaret Farley expresses a similar concern, arguing that theories of relativity preclude the possibility of "a common cry for justice" among women.[2] In order to speak meaningfully about human purposes and goals, as well as to combat the myriad horrors committed against women in the name of social tradition and particularity, what is needed is a thoughtful, careful, and critical moral realism, one that reflects broadly on human "nature" and experience even while appreciating and valuing human difference.

The goal here is not a final, unchangeable list of what it means to flourish as a human being, a woman, or as a parent or child; rather, the task is to begin to articulate provisional ideas about how human beings function best, individually, socially, and, for purposes of the present work, in parent-child relations. It should be emphasized here that any such ideas will indeed be *provisional.* Our visions of human flourishing must walk a fine line between tentativeness and absolutism, yielding normative claims with enough moral muscle to foster human liberation, but also remaining cognizant of the cultural pluralism and historical change that distinctively mark our human situation.[3] What I put forth in this chapter is a preliminary effort to specify which forms of genetic manipulation are most likely to foster integral human flourishing, and which are most likely to contradict it. My account is necessarily limited and therefore functions in part as a call for critique and dialogue, particularly by others from different social, cultural, and geographic locations. In spite of this provisionality, however, it is my belief that many of the qualities that I put forth in this chapter to specify a normative vision of procreation and family life do indeed have widespread appeal and begin to shape a picture of what might be considered genuine integral human flourishing in these contexts.

Careful reflection on human experience does begin to yield certain insights about what it means to flourish as a human being, and more particularly to flourish in parent-child relationships. This is not to say that every human individual will do best when her or his life reflects these ideals, much less that these ideals provide a sufficient account of what it means to live well in any given case. Rather, such thoughtful reflection aims at sketching some broad outlines of a good human life, outlines that might reasonably be expected to accord with widely shared values. When a life (or the shared life of a group of people) radically departs from such guidelines, we are right to question whether human well-being is served.

From a Christian perspective, such a broad articulation of human flourishing might be said to reflect divine intention for human life. The Christian God wills human well-being and, more broadly, the well-being of all creation. The particular Christian approach advocated in this book is that this divine intent includes, but is not limited to, truths that are revealed by way of biology or physical reality — that which is often simply referred to as the "natural." Certainly we must avoid a narrowly physicalist approach that undervalues the role of human reason and avoids any ongoing human responsibility for co-creation.[4] Yet Christianity, in my view, also will not allow us to ignore entirely the good that *is* — in other words, the good that is manifest in nature itself and that we may too quickly look past in an effort to shape and control our experiences of the world. Part of the task of Christian moral theology must be to work out the parameters of God's intentions, searching human experience deeply and reflecting carefully on that experience in light of Christian faith in order to begin to name what is normative for human beings — that is, what God intends.

Further, a distinctively Christian approach will be marked by a spirit of hopefulness, not fear. As I argued in the previous chapter, part of what should characterize a Christian moral posture is an optimism about our possibilities as partners with God in the creative process, for the Christian God is fundamentally one who empowers human beings to help create a better world. Certainly, Christian faith also calls us to a keen awareness of human sin and its insidious power over us, and we do well to keep this in mind as we take steps to specify which interventions truly foster human well-being. Yet the goal of specifying certain components of human flourishing is not primarily to restrain us from acting on our growing technological abilities, though that will at times be necessary; rather, it is to help guide us in making creative use of these abilities in the service of human well-being.

Finally, a Christian approach must include a commitment to support God's "preferential option" for the poor, or, more broadly, the societally marginalized. In the case of genetic manipulation this will include attention to social justice, such that genetic manipulation does not reinforce the social and economic marginalization of the poor or the otherwise disenfranchised, or inadvertently reduce a "good" diversity in the name of promoting individual control and choice. A feminist Christian approach also includes a warrant to focus on and support specifically the well-being of women and children, who, as I have argued, have historically possessed limited social power in the realm of reproductive matters. The account presented here will seek to remain attentive to these tasks.

Visions of Human Flourishing

Contributing Perspectives on Human Well-Being

A few years ago, Bill Watterson's *Calvin and Hobbes* comic strip portrayed the strip's main character, a small boy named Calvin, having an ad hoc philosophical discussion with his friend and confidant, a stuffed toy tiger named Hobbes. Hobbes is asking Calvin about his New Year's resolutions, to which Calvin replies that he did not make any. "See," Calvin explains earnestly, "in order to improve oneself, one must have some idea of what's 'Good.' That implies certain values. But as we all know, values are relative. Every system of belief is equally valid and we need to tolerate diversity. Virtue isn't 'better' than vice. It's just different." Hobbes, looking somewhat nonplused, answers simply, "I don't know if I can tolerate that much tolerance."

Keeping company with Hobbes, we should not allow an admirable desire to tolerate a diversity of perspectives to keep us from articulating what exactly is good and worthy in human existence. A resurgence of interest in Aristotelian virtue theory over the past few years has prompted many Christians and non-Christians alike to try to do just that: to name what is basic to human well-being. It would be impossible (and likely not very helpful here) to survey these in any sort of depth or completeness. Instead, I will draw on the work of a few key thinkers in the course of shaping my own picture of what human flourishing looks like with respect to human procreation, particularly as it is changed, and challenged, by genetic manipulation.

An Integral View of Human Flourishing

The goal of an adequate account of human well-being should be to weave together both physical and nonphysical aspects into what Christina Traina has called an "integral" picture of human flourishing — encompassing the various dimensions of a "good" human life, and where no dimension of human well-being is sacrificed permanently in the service of others.[5] Again, as we examine the implications of genetic manipulation, we cannot ignore or deride (for instance) its emotional impact on women simply because it may support the feminist goal of reproductive freedom; nor can we disregard the ways that particular forms of genetic manipulation may support or threaten the well-being of children simply because we wish to uphold the integrity of a parent's personal choice.

I will structure my own picture of human flourishing — a feminist Christian picture — in terms of four primary components of human well-being: physical, emotional, relational, and social — all of which are, of course, interrelated. My goal here is not to describe human flourishing exhaustively; rather, I will focus especially on the aspects most likely to be directly affected by the possibilities of genetic manipulation. This will pave the way for later analysis of the three specific cases of genetic manipulation under discussion here.

Physical Well-Being

Before all else, a holistic view of human flourishing, if it is to remain faithful to the concept of human embodiment, must include attention to persons' bodily well-being and other physical needs. Here the work of philosopher Martha Nussbaum is particularly helpful. Nussbaum has attempted to work out what she calls a "critical universalism" that tries to assess human, and specifically women's, well-being across gaps in history and culture. Working with the "capabilities approach" pioneered by economist Amartya Sen, Nussbaum focuses on human capabilities for functioning well in the world. Seeking to remain sensitive and open to historical and cultural differences, she nevertheless boldly lists, first, the "shape" of, and the forms of "activity" distinctive to, human life;[6] and, second, eleven "basic functional capabilities at which societies should aim for their citizens" and without which a human life cannot be considered "good."[7]

It is this second list that is of particular use here, since it attempts to outline the capabilities necessary for human flourishing. It is comprised of the following capabilities:

1. to live a human life of normal length;
2. to have good health and adequate nourishment, shelter, opportunities for sexual satisfaction, choice in reproductive matters, and mobility;
3. to avoid unnecessary and nonbeneficial pain (so far as possible) and to have pleasurable experiences;
4. to use the senses, to imagine, think and reason, all informed by adequate education;
5. to have attachments to things and persons outside of oneself;
6. to form a conception of the good and engage in critical reflection about the planning of one's own life;
7. to show concern for others;

8. to live with concern for and in relation to animals, plants, and nature;
9. to laugh, play, and enjoy recreational activities;
10. to live one's own life with a guarantee of some noninterference with certain personal choices that are definitive of selfhood (e.g., marriage, childbearing, sexual expression, speech, employment);
11. to live one's own life in one's own surroundings and context — that is, to enjoy freedom of association, freedom from unwarranted search and seizure, and, to a degree, the integrity of personal property.[8]

Within this list we may highlight the sheer length of life as well as varied aspects of physical well-being, including good health, nourishment, shelter, mobility, sexual satisfaction, the elimination of nonbeneficial pain, and the ability to enjoy some sort of recreational activity. These criteria are, of course, somewhat relative to time and place; life expectancy, for instance, has risen dramatically in much of the world even over the past half century. Still, in every time and place it seems likely that reasonable people could achieve *some* consensus on the general parameters of life's length, so that diseases that threaten to acutely foreshorten a life could be considered to contradict human flourishing. That is not to say that such a foreshortened life would not be worth living at all; rather, we can specify that societies generally should set as a goal a reasonable life expectancy for each person.

Similarly, good health itself may be considered a rather slippery concept. The World Health Organization's definition of health ("a state of complete physical, mental and social well-being, and not merely the absence of disease or infirmity"[9]) is so broad as to be functionally useless in many specific cases of shaping policy. Moreover, as proponents for the disabled community have reminded us, what is considered "healthy" often depends heavily on social context and expectation. Deafness, for example, is a much greater "disability" in a society in which only a very few people use sign language. Yet again it seems likely that some degree of consensus could be reached about conditions that clearly contradict good health. For instance, it seems apparent that certain severe genetic disorders — one of the clearest cases would be Tay Sachs disease, a degenerative disease of the central nervous system that leads to blindness, paralysis, unawareness of one's surroundings, and death by age five — would significantly hinder even a minimal level of health and recreational enjoyment.

Nussbaum's description of this sort of physical well-being, of course, echoes many of the feminist concerns outlined in chapter 3. Hence, as we examine genetic technologies more specifically, we can safely insist that any such technologies must be shown to be safe for the women on whose bodies they are performed and for the children who are affected by them. To ignore or soft-pedal these considerations would constitute an unacceptable contradiction to the well-being of women and children.

A Christian analysis, as described in chapter 4, adds the strong injunction that part of our human responsibility toward one another is to make use of our powers to reduce suffering and to *heal.* This, along with Nussbaum's criteria, fortifies the conviction that genetic manipulations are relatively more acceptable when they are designed to rectify conditions that significantly foreshorten life span or when they aim to reduce or prevent nonbeneficial pain (Nussbaum's term) and human suffering — especially severe suffering that threatens or makes impossible some baseline level of overall health, nourishment, mobility, and so on. Again, I do not wish to argue that a life devoid of, say, mobility (e.g., when a person is completely paralyzed) is not a life worth living; rather, when genetic manipulation could be employed to correct or prevent such severe disability, we may in fact have an obligation to do so. There is enormous promise in the advance of genetic technologies, promise for reducing childhood pain, suffering, and premature death. It is essential not to overlook this promise even while pointing out the many troublesome pitfalls that the advent of genetic manipulation introduces. Indeed, Christian faith instructs us that part of our human calling is to act in a spirit of hopefulness to help further the work of God, including especially the *healing* work of God.

Emotional Well-Being

It is not enough simply to concern ourselves with the effects of genetic manipulation on physical health and well-being; we also must look more broadly, to emotional and social/relational well-being. Of course, Nussbaum's category of flourishing that includes the capability to laugh, play, and enjoy recreational activities expresses not only an element of physical well-being, but also emotional well-being. That is, the ability to enjoy life in these ways is an essential part of our emotional flourishing. In order to promote the well-being of the whole person, then, we must discourage genetic practices that might artificially limit these recreational possibilities — for instance, the intentional diminishment that strong liberals (e.g., John Robertson) sometimes seem to sanction.

Beyond this, it is instructive to turn to the category of intimate family relations to describe what we mean by emotional flourishing. Nussbaum's fifth category includes the abilities to love, to grieve, and to experience longing and gratitude. Significantly, this includes the capability for some form of intimate family love, though in her view this need not take the form of the traditional Western nuclear family.[10] As I have argued in previous chapters, the prospect of genetic manipulation could affect, however subtly, the way we as a society, and as parents and potential parents, understand parent-child bonds, so that control and choice rise in prominence relative to love and affection. Again, Nussbaum's category highlights that such a change in understanding is not insignificant, but rather ultimately contradicts human well-being.

Christian tradition, as described in this book, has something to add about the quality of family relations in regard to emotional flourishing. According to the general understanding of Christian ethicists, children by their very existence merit, and flourish best when offered, our unconditional love and basic acceptance. If parents are discouraged from first accepting and loving their children in the midst of frailty and imperfection, before trying to nurture their growth and development in specific directions, something important is in danger of being lost, both in the parental vocation itself and in the likely well-being of the child.

Parents must recognize that their children are akin to gifts entrusted to their care by God, not possessions to be molded according to personal desire or whim. This recognition itself is part of what it means to flourish in the role of parent: to open oneself to the unexpected beauty of the child who is before us. Children, for their part, must be able to trust that parents will not fail to recognize their basic dignity, beauty, and goodness in a too hasty effort to mold and shape their development.

These insights go hand-in-hand with the astute reflections of bioethicist Thomas Murray. Murray pushes a step further than Nussbaum by describing in more detail what intimate family love implies. First, he is clear that individualism and marketplace values are a poor foundation on which to build a healthy understanding of children and families. He lambastes those who uncritically celebrate individual choice, control, and commercialization at the expense of other values. In his view, these concepts simply do not capture what most of us recognize is particularly valuable about families.

Part of the danger, in Murray's view, is that if we begin to regard children as "carefully and willfully" produced, we may begin to think of the parent-child bond as resembling an acquisition-like relationship rather than a bond of biology, custom, or law between actual vulnerable human beings. Inevitably this will lead to disappointment, as our all-too-human children fail to live up to our expectations. If children are objects of conscious manipulation, parents may become less tolerant of imperfection and more likely to feel a heightened sense of responsibility and guilt for a child's inevitable shortcomings; this guilt in turn may impede the love and acceptance necessary for a child to develop maturity and self-confidence. In this way, "the quest for the perfect child can create an environment hostile to children — and adults — as they are, with their many imperfections."[11] Furthermore, our social institutions may in turn come to reflect this lack of acceptance and forgiveness, showing decreasing support for children with disabilities.

Murray feels that, above all, families should serve the values of love, loyalty, affection, forgiveness, trust, care, nurturing, maturation, identity, and self-confidence.[12] He acknowledges that this is a "partial list" of what characterizes healthy families, but he insists that it will be broadly recognizable to most late-twentieth-century Americans and perhaps even to those in different times and cultures. Implied in these values, he indicates, are acceptance over and above control, and the honoring of unchosen obligations over and above individual choice. It is not that choice and control are intrinsically disvaluable or have no role at all within families; rather, they should not be considered the central aspect of family life. Given the sort of creatures that we humans are, these values are simply not well-suited to support the flourishing of children and adults within families. Unlike the marketplace, the family rightly centers on nurturing relationships, not choice and control.

Very often, Murray points out, this commitment to nurture relationships entails an acceptance of imperfection on the part of parents. In other words, the meaning of parenthood for human beings should include the development and nurture of the parent-child bond in the face of our (and our children's) sometimes painful human shortcomings. Thus, rejecting "perfectibilism," we can "embrace a conception of parenthood as the sustained effort to work out unmistakably human relationships, that is, relationships devoted to fostering love, dedication, and mutuality, in the face of ever-present imperfection, ambivalence, and disappointment."[13] To espouse such a view is to properly understand what a family *is*, at its heart, as well as the rightful place of children in family life.

Murray's central point here is that the tendency to view children primarily as objects to be both owned and perfected impedes the love and acceptance necessary for a child to attain self-assurance and develop a healthy identity. Children as well as adults must be able to trust that their families will provide a sustained environment in which they are loved and accepted for who they are, not simply for who or what they can become. This indeed is part and parcel of what we treasure about families, and it is an important part of human flourishing. Hence, acceptance, love, affection, and care are indispensable in the raising of children, and we must be supremely careful of embracing, even unwittingly, a concept of parenting whereby these play only a secondary role.

This means, above all, that we should resist forms of genetic manipulation that express an unduly perfectionist mindset and the desire to shape and control children rather than to nurture and love them. Although it is incumbent upon parents to attend to their children's well-being, parents also must be careful not to misplace their hopes and aspirations, interpreting this mandate as an excuse for adopting a perfectionist or control-oriented mindset that fails to see and honor the flowering of an actual child.

Feminist commitments demand that we raise a similar concern about the emotional well-being of children, including the impact on an individual child of knowing that he or she was (or was not) genetically manipulated. For example, what would the experience be like for a child to grow up in the world knowing that he was chosen to be a boy, and perhaps a firstborn boy, designed to have a better-than-average memory (and thus, in the hopes of his parents, highly intelligent)? Again, it seems quite likely that such a child could experience an undue and unhealthy sense of pressure to achieve the expectations that have been set for him even before his birth. Similarly, a child who has been "chosen" to be a girl — say, so that a mother could satisfy her own unfulfilled desires for professional achievement in and through her daughter — would likely experience quite a heavy burden of expectation to be someone other than who she may be personally inclined to be. Furthermore, a child who is *not* genetically engineered, and knows it, may wonder about "measuring up" in a world where he or she perceives that other children have a distinct, genetically manipulated advantage. Feminism instructs us not to ignore the dangers that these scenarios present. Children's well-being certainly is not enhanced by this sort of pressure and objectification. Although perhaps no child grows up free of all unwarranted parental and social expectations, it seems likely that genetic manipulation may exacerbate such expectations immensely, closing off a child's sense of openness about his or her life.

The possibilities presented by genetic manipulation cause us to look not only to the emotional well-being of children, to be sure, but also to the emotional flourishing of the women whose bodies will very likely be the locus for the implementation of these technologies. Again, with feminism as our guide, it is crucial to remember that women's emotional well-being is bound up with the public conception of them as more than simply reproductive "machines." To the degree that society sustains a view of women as "breeders," identifiable with their reproductive capacities, women are harmed, individually and collectively. They may come to see themselves this way, or they may simply be forced to interact with a world where their nonreproductive selves are neglected or otherwise subtly devalued. In either case, human flourishing is not well-served. A feminist understanding of well-being must be especially wary of genetic manipulations that may exacerbate these harmful tendencies.

Relational Well-Being

The relational dimensions of human flourishing are deeply connected, of course, to many of the emotional aspects already considered. It is destructive to think of human well-being apart from relational well-being. Relational well-being, according to the feminist patterns of analysis embraced here, includes first and foremost an emphasis on the basic social equality of men and women. Such social equality not only translates into concrete socioeconomic parity (such as equal access to employment opportunities or equal responsibility for childcare arrangements), but also encompasses the more intangible social *perceptions* of men and women that might be affected by our particular social arrangements and practices. Hence, genetic manipulations that, when widely implemented, threaten to exacerbate existing trends of socioeconomic inequality between men and women must be challenged, and so must those that threaten to entrench harmful social perceptions of the relative worth of women and men. Indeed, any genetic technology that potentially endangers on any level the basic social equality between women and men must remain highly suspect, and such interventions would need to be justified by very strong countervailing arguments.

On a more interpersonal level, feminism's advocacy of mutuality informs our portrait of relational well-being. In other words, human beings flourish best when they relate in patterns of reciprocity, cooperation, and mutual respect rather than those marked by domination and submission. Murray too embraces this point when he lists mutuality, along with love and dedication, as a hallmark value that parents should strive to foster in their families.[14] In the context of families, mutuality itself translates into an atmosphere wherein children are treated not as a particularly valuable form of property, but rather are supported and nurtured as the potentially autonomous, and yet deeply relational, beings that they are. This again points toward a rejection of genetic manipulations that seem to encourage a highly possessive and perfectionist attitude in parents toward their children.

Mutuality also has another, less straightforward, implication. The value of mutuality would seem to suggest a less individualized and more shared, even collective, responsibility for the well-being of children. That is, instead of individual parents — in today's world, usually mothers — shouldering the primary responsibility for children's upbringing, mutuality suggests that fathers and even the wider community collaborate to nurture children and foster their development. It is possible that widespread use of genetic manipulation could lead to a scenario whereby parents — again, particularly mothers — experience a heightened sense of responsibility not only for a child's upbringing, but also for his or her genetic makeup. Rather than fostering the sense that the joys and strains of childrearing may and should be shared, such a trend could in fact leave parents increasingly isolated in reproductive matters. This is especially troublesome when a particular child — for instance, one with an unforeseen birth "defect" — requires special amounts of time and attention.

It is, of course, difficult to gauge the likelihood of such a trend occurring, and it is impossible to isolate any particular forms of genetic manipulation that would be more or less likely to bring about such a subtle change in sensibilities. Yet here again we can say that the danger itself should lead us to require very good reasons for any genetic manipulations that we do allow. If society is to support mutuality as a value conducive to human well-being, it must guard against these sorts of subtle changes that potentially isolate parents rather than bringing them into more fully cooperative relations in their childrearing responsibilities.

The distinctively Christian contribution to relational well-being is closely bound up with Christian insights about parent-child relations and socioeconomic justice. Yet Christianity also adds the insight that human flourishing depends in part upon the responsible and thoughtful acceptance of our place in the cosmos, including the careful exercise of our human freedom. That is, our "relational" well-being depends not simply on our proper relatedness to each other, but also on the acceptance of our "place" in the universe, before God. God has created us to be free and yet also *discerning* — discerning of how best to use that freedom in order to promote God's purposes for creation.

Hence, genetic manipulation should be embraced only in a way that takes seriously this need for careful discernment. From a Christian perspective, unrestrained advocacy for genetic manipulation, even in the name of human freedom, is unwarranted, for it fails to consider its many and varied pitfalls of genetic manipulation and may pander to an overdeveloped sense of human control over nature. On the other hand, complete disregard for the hopeful possibilities that genetic manipulation offers would also be an unfaithful response, evading our co-creative responsibilities. If human beings are to flourish in their relation to God vis-à-vis genetic technology, we must disavow both a fearful rejection of genetic manipulation and a wholehearted embrace of it; rather, we should maintain something more akin to Rahner's "cool-headedness" and seek to discern carefully the ways in which genetic technology may serve God's purposes (including human well-being) as well as the ways in which it contradicts them.

Social Well-Being

Finally, as should be clear by this point, relational well-being necessarily includes attention to the broader socioeconomic relations in which persons are embedded. These are part of what Christianity tends to refer to as the common good. Thus, we must not only look to issues of social equality between men and women; we must also attend to the categories of social diversity, on the one hand, and economic justice, on the other. Turning first to diversity, we must grant that diversity is not of unlimited value; there are harmful conditions that certainly should not be protected in its name. Yet there is merit in what might be considered a "good" diversity — one wherein persons are basically valued for their God-given uniqueness, and differences generally are not leveled out, but rather are dealt with constructively and creatively. Minimally, upholding this kind of diversity means welcoming differences of gender and skin color; it also means that generally we will resist flattening out the human array of intellectual abilities, personalities, and body types. Indeed, it is my contention that to flourish as human beings, we must live in a society that upholds diversity in these ways. In other words, we do better as people when we learn from and work with our differences; our horizons are broadened. Again, this does not mean that any human circumstance, even those that seem harmful, must be accepted in the name of human diversity. It does mean, however, that we are right to challenge genetic manipulations that would move our society toward a more homogenous (less diverse) population (racially, sexually, or even in terms of intelligence, body type, personality, and so on) without very good cause. Genetic enhancement presents a particularly troubling scenario, for what counts at any given time as "enhancement" would more than likely reflect ephemeral social preferences rather than the true best interests of persons or of society as a whole. We must be guided by a strong commitment to upholding human social diversity in the face of individual preferences that may collectively lead us otherwise.

Hand-in-hand with a commitment to honoring human social diversity goes a mandate to support some degree of equitable sharing and to foster economic justice in the public realm. The feminist Christian vision that I have advocated here is opposed to severe socioeconomic inequality; indeed, feminism and Christianity both hold that humans generally do not flourish in societies that are marked by such inequality. To the degree that genetic manipulation aggravates these inequalities by offering the financially well-off yet another means of "getting ahead," while leaving the poorer segments of society no better off than they were before, these technologies must be resisted. In other words, the genetic manipulation of offspring must not be used to create a society of genetic "haves" and "have-nots." If the genetic manipulation of offspring is to be supported in any form, it must be made available even to those who cannot pay for it themselves and who are less likely to have access to health insurance that might cover it for them. That is, its gains must be distributed to all.

Of course, the question remains, from the standpoint of socio-economic justice, whether or not scarce healthcare dollars should be utilized in the service of genetic manipulation at all — a point that has been touched on above. If societies are to flourish, other, more pressing, low-tech healthcare concerns must not be ignored. Basic healthcare must be provided for all (a goal that we in the United States are nowhere near achieving), and steps must be taken to address public health concerns that currently contribute to the immense gap in health between the poor and the rich — concerns including, for instance, poor housing and homelessness, malnutrition, chronic stress, and substandard working conditions.[15] If these concerns are ignored, there is little justification that may be found, from a feminist Christian standpoint, for society to encourage the high-tech prospects of genetic manipulation, which, relative to these other measures, would aid comparatively few people. This is especially true for genetic interventions that do not directly address health and disease at all, and that, in the context of widespread poverty and poverty-related illness, seem an ill-afforded luxury.

Even in the context of all these social and relational considerations, many of which appear to work against support for genetic manipulation, it is important to reaffirm that the feminist Christian perspective that I am putting forth here does not deny that some level of reproductive freedom is essential to human, and especially women's, well-being. Within the concrete context of human history, particularly in the United States, reproductive freedom represents a recognition that women too are full moral agents and must be respected as such. It also represents the acknowledgment that women's concrete bodily and social well-being has depended, and does still depend, on some guarantee of control over their reproductive lives. From a Christian perspective, reproductive freedom may be considered as one manifestation of responsible human co-creativity, one way in which human beings are called to make use of their freedom to serve divine purposes. It is not my intent to exclude reproductive freedom from an account of human flourishing; indeed, to cast off the concept altogether would be enormously harmful to women (and, indeed, to all parents), would violate their status as full moral agents, and would in fact be to shy away from the immense responsibilities that God has given human beings.

Indeed, here it is important to highlight the impact of another of Nussbaum's contributors to human flourishing: the ability to "live one's own life and no one else's." This capability calls for guarantees against interference in certain "especially personal" choices that are "definitive of selfhood" (including choices regarding marriage and childbearing). Nussbaum does not go into great detail here about precisely what constitutes such protected choices or what are their limits. Moreover, it is evident that a "choice" that is "definitive of selfhood" in one society (e.g., the individual choice of a marriage partner) may not seem so in another (a society that adheres to the custom of family-arranged marriages). Even if we grant that some degree of variation can exist, however, it seems reasonable to expect that some minimal level of protected personal choice in these arenas could indeed be considered basic to human well-being.

Here we must be careful neither to assume that the relatively high level of choice commonly expected in U.S. society is normative for all societies, nor to slip into a relativist, "anything goes" approach wherein everything depends entirely on the individual's self-understanding and choice of priorities and values. Again, certain choices will remain personal enough to be protected against interference in every time and place. What those are is up for debate. It seems clear, however, that the choice to predetermine a child's memory, intelligence level, hair or eye color, and so on can hardly be considered a choice that is "definitive of selfhood," at least from a Christian perspective as it has been outlined in this book. Even those not operating from Christian assumptions will be hard-pressed in today's world to argue that such choices are definitive of selfhood. Choices regarding health (and disease) and sex selection may be less clear, for some may argue that these indeed are more often closely connected to a sense of self. Yet even here, it is important to ask whether it is appropriate in the first place for a parent to link her or his own self-definition with the health or gender of offspring. Indeed, from the perspective of the child-to-be, such decisions may be perceived as a violation of his or her own integrity and selfhood. In any case, it is not at all clear that the choice of what *kind* of child to have (i.e., the choice to shape one's offspring genetically) falls into any category of personal choice that can broadly be considered "definitive of selfhood."

Still, in general terms, we can affirm that reproductive freedom exists as one very important aspect of human flourishing. What I am arguing in this chapter, however, is that human flourishing, even procreative flourishing, is in fact much broader than the concept of reproductive freedom by itself suggests. If reproductive freedom is truly to serve human well-being, it must be situated into the context of the integral flourishing of persons, understood as bodily, emotional, relational, and social human beings. This means that at times human flourishing will require that procreative liberty be curtailed, and that society act to discourage individuals from exercising it where it seems that its exercise in the short term will threaten longer-term human welfare.

Notes

1. C. S. Lewis, *The Abolition of Man* (New York: Touchstone, 1944), 74.
2. Christina L. H. Traina, *Feminist Ethics and Natural Law: The End of Anathemas* (Washington, D.C.: Georgetown University Press, 1999), 35, citing Susan Frank Parsons, *Feminism and Christian Ethics* (Cambridge: Cambridge University Press, 1996), 108; Margaret A. Farley, "Feminism and Universal Morality," in *Prospects for a Common Morality*, ed. Gene Outka and John P. Reeder Jr. (Princeton, N.J.: Princeton University Press, 1993), 178.
3. Traina, *Feminist Ethics and Natural Law*, 43.
4. See Maura A. Ryan, "Feminist Theology and the New Genetics," in *The Ethics of Genetic Engineering*, ed. Maureen Junker-Kenny and Lisa Sowle Cahill (London: SCM Press, 1998), 100.
5. Traina, *Feminist Ethics and Natural Law*, 44, 46.

6. This list includes the following: mortality; a distinctive human body with associated bodily needs; the capacity for pleasure and pain; the cognitive capabilities of perceiving, imagining, and thinking; early infant development; the capacity for practical reason; affiliation with other human beings; relatedness to other species and to nature; humor and play; separateness; and contextual particularity. See Martha C. Nussbaum, "Human Capabilities, Female Human Beings," in *Women, Culture and Development: A Study of Human Capabilities,* ed. Martha Nussbaum and Jonathan Glover (New York: Oxford University Press, 1995), 76–80.

7. Ibid., 82, 85.

8. Ibid., 83–85.

9. Gilbert Meilaender, *Bioethics: A Primer for Christians* (Grand Rapids: Eerdmans, 1996), 44.

10. Nussbaum "Human Capabilities, Female Human Beings," 84 n. 55.

11. Thomas Murray, *The Worth of a Child* (Berkeley: University of California Press, 1996), 12.

12. Ibid., 23–24.

13. Ibid., 136.

14. Ibid.

15. See Suzanne Holland and Karen Peterson, "The Health Care *Titanic:* Women and Children First?" *Second Opinion* 18, no. 3 (1993): 11–13; Lorna McBarnette, "Women and Poverty: The Effects on Reproductive Status," in *Too Little, Too Late: Dealing with the Health Needs of Women in Poverty,* ed. Cesar A. Perales and Lauren S. Young (New York: Harrington, 1988), 55–81; Ruth E. Zambrana, "A Research Agenda on Issues Affecting Poor and Minority Women: A Model for Understanding Their Health Needs," in Perales and Young, eds., *Too Little, Too Late,* 137–60.

Chapter Six

The Limits of Genetic Control

After all, what parent would really want to shape and determine absolutely a child's personality? To reach for certainties, for Nature or Nurture, is to look right past the joy of raising children, the comedy and the tragedy of it, and above all, the all-consuming interest of it.

— PERRI KLASS[1]

TO THIS POINT, I have painted a partial picture of integral human flourishing, especially procreative flourishing, that seeks to adhere to the feminist and Christian insights embraced in this book. Human well-being, especially in the context of procreative relations, requires attention to physical, emotional, relational, and social well-being. It not only requires that we protect human freedom and physical health and life, but also entails careful attention to how people perceive themselves and are perceived by the rest of society, and to the quality of relations that exist between women and men, between parents and children, between children and the rest of society, and between various social groups. None of these considerations may be ignored if we are to attend to the well-being of human beings as they truly exist in the world.

I return now to how this vision of human flourishing affects our evaluation of the specific sorts of genetic manipulation presented in the first chapter of this book. I will examine each type of genetic manipulation in turn, recognizing that many of the insights brought up in the analyses will overlap.

Disease Prevention as Design: The Case of Cystic Fibrosis

Examining Arguments against Genetic Manipulation

In some ways, genetic manipulation undertaken to prevent cystic fibrosis (CF) in a child at risk for the disease is the easiest of the cases under analysis here. The comparatively serious nature of CF, the physical and emotional strain that it places on individuals and families, and its relatively common occurrence in the population all combine to make it a genuine threat to human well-being and hence an attractive candidate for gene therapy. Still, there are several factors that mitigate the straightforward acceptance of genetic manipulation to prevent CF. First, there is a fairly wide range in the severity of CF cases. Although the average life expectancy of a person with CF is about thirty-three years, some people with milder cases manage to live reasonably normal lives and do not die at an inordinately young age. Hence, the element of human flourishing that Nussbaum articulates as the capability to live a life of "normal" length may be violated to a relatively greater or lesser extent, depending on the severity of any given case of CF — something that parents presumably could not know in advance. Second, as noted in chapter 1, there are several promising drug treatments available for CF patients, so that the more elaborate measures involving gene therapy or, further down the line, preventive genetic manipulation could be considered a superfluous expenditure of money and energy.

Third, and perhaps most importantly, the physical dangers inherent in the development of any form of genetic manipulation, including this one, are great. The 1999 death of eighteen-year-old gene therapy patient Jesse Gelsinger made headline news, in part because Jesse himself suffered not from a life-threatening disorder, but rather from a relatively less serious form of an enzyme deficiency: ornithine transcarbamylase (OTC) deficiency. In patients with OTC deficiency the liver cannot process ammonia, a toxin released as the body breaks down food. Jesse's particular form of the condition was treatable through drugs and dietary measures, but he participated in a gene therapy experiment designed to benefit infants with a fatal form of the disorder. His subsequent death, due to a severe and unforeseen immune response, provoked the U.S. Food and Drug Administration to shut down all gene therapy experiments at the University of Pennsylvania, where his study was carried out, and to monitor more closely all clinical trials involving gene therapy generally.[2]

The case of Jesse Gelsinger serves to highlight the myriad safety issues that genetic manipulation presents. It raises questions not only about the adequacy of informed-consent requirements and procedures, but also about how accurately researchers can foresee the risks entailed by a procedure and how eager, or even willing, they are to reveal those risks to volunteers.[3] Ruth Macklin, a bioethicist on the National Institutes of Health Recombinant DNA Advisory Committee (RAC), points out that many researchers involved in gene therapy have a large financial stake in the success of the experiments, a fact that should provoke doubts about their ability to adequately carry out informed-consent measures designed to protect patients. A Christian account, wary of tendencies toward human sin (including relatively unwitting forms of human sin), will not ignore this danger, for it represents an instance where self-interest may cloud researchers' better judgment. Of course, even if informed-consent procedures are strictly adhered to, there lingers the bare fact that gene therapy is still in a highly experimental stage and inevitably engenders serious safety concerns, concerns that researchers are still a long, long way from overcoming. Thus, before becoming overly sanguine about the present and future possibilities of genetic manipulation, we are wise to pause and remind ourselves of the grave physical dangers that realizing those possibilities will entail. Furthermore, as we move from gene therapy to proactive genetic manipulation (i.e., on embryos or gametes), those physical dangers will disproportionately affect women because women's bodies will be the likely locus of intervention. From a feminist standpoint, this is troublesome.

Beyond the immediate physical dangers inherent in this and other forms of genetic manipulation, the genetic prevention of CF introduces some of the other concerns mentioned earlier. For example, absent significant healthcare reform measures, we can predict with relative accuracy that such treatment will not be equally available to patients with differential access to the current healthcare system; hence, it is likely disproportionately to benefit financially well-off families and, in so doing, may indeed foster a social split between the genetic "haves" and "have-nots." Moreover, as increasing numbers of wealthy or middle-class families are more able to take advantage of the technology, social acceptance may fall for families with CF-disabled children, leading to even further social isolation for those of lesser financial means. On the other hand, in order to choose to prioritize this sort of genetic treatment such that it is made available to all, regardless of ability to pay, society would need to funnel resources away from other, less costly, low-tech healthcare measures, measures that likely would affect the health of a far greater portion of the overall population, including especially the poor.[4] Again, to advocate a "preferential option" for the poor requires that we not ignore these considerations.

Finally, there is the concern, raised frequently by advocates for persons with disabilities, that technological measures such as genetic manipulation for the prevention of CF subtly encourage the view that persons with disabilities are of lesser worth. Furthermore, the argument goes, disability itself is heavily socially constructed, and it is incumbent on society to make the necessary alterations so that persons of all body types, including persons with disabilities, are included in mainstream social life. Those who embrace this view tend to reject or resist gene therapy in all its forms. This is the argument for diversity taken to an extreme position; here, even physical "dysfunction" is defended in the name of human difference.

This view, in spite of its merits, does not seem true to the ordinary human experience of illness, disability, and disease. Acknowledging the equal worth of all persons, including those with disabilities, does not mean that we need to embrace the existence of those disabilities themselves. In other words, we may consider persons with CF to be no less valuable as persons and still wish, for their sake, that they did not suffer the dysfunction associated with CF. As I have argued, a feminist Christian view must embrace the value of human diversity; yet CF, according to the understanding of human flourishing promoted here, should not be considered part of any "good" diversity.

In spite of this final qualifier, most of the aforementioned factors appear to challenge our immediate acceptance of genetic manipulation for the prevention of CF, at least at first glance. Not only is physical human flourishing seemingly threatened by this technology, but so also is the common good that is manifested in terms of socioeconomic equality with respect to healthcare. In other words, we are in danger of aggravating existing social inequalities through our use of genetic means. Furthermore, unless society significantly increases the allotment of public funds toward basic healthcare, it appears that the public financing of this form of genetic manipulation would result in a decreased emphasis on more low-tech measures, measures that would significantly aid less financially secure people by extending them guaranteed access to basic healthcare. Finally, even if we refuse to accept the existence of CF as a part of a "good" diversity, we as a society will have to take care not to allow this form of genetic manipulation subtly to translate into a social intolerance toward *people* with CF. These concerns are serious ones, but there are also arguments on the other side of the equation, arguments that persuade strongly toward the acceptance of genetic manipulation for the prevention of CF.

Examining Arguments for Genetic Manipulation

The most important of these argument for genetic manipulation in the case of CF is that the potential gains for CF patients are enormous. For a disease that threatens the basic health and life of many of those who suffer from it, that limits their opportunities for physical comfort and recreation, and that places a severe emotional strain on them and their families, the hope offered by genetic manipulation must not be underestimated. According to the view of human flourishing that I have constructed, the lives of many (albeit not all) CF patients fall far short of what we might consider to comprise basic well-being. If the technology could be made safe for the children and women most directly affected by it, it could offer immense hope to families that otherwise face the possibility of a fairly bleak future. A feminist and Christian account devoted to promoting human well-being and neighbor-love must not downplay this prospect.

What of the other concerns raised, concerns related to the emotional and relational well-being of the women and children most directly affected by any form of genetic manipulation, including this one? First we must consider the emotional impact on a child of knowing that she or he was genetically "engineered" so as not to suffer the effects of CF. As noted in earlier chapters, it is difficult to envision that such a child would experience any sense of not being fundamentally accepted, or a related lack of self-confidence. There would most likely not be heightened pressures or expectations placed upon that child beyond simply respecting her or his own life and health. Because the conditions associated with CF so clearly violate my account of basic human well-being, and because it is generally accepted in our society that having a disease as serious as CF has an overall negative impact on one's life, it is most likely that a child who has been genetically manipulated not to have CF will be pleased, not resentful, at the resulting state of health.

Here again the distinction between the normal and the abnormal comes into play. The view of human well-being embraced here assumes that such a distinction can be made and that it is not entirely socially constructed. In other words, there are realities about health and disease that transcend culture, such that certain disorders can be said to contradict human flourishing regardless of time and place. CF appears to be one of those disorders. Its debilitating nature depends heavily on its physical impact and not, primarily, on social or cultural interpretation. Certainly, social construction will play some role; a serious case of CF that severely limits independence no doubt will be interpreted as comparatively more problematic in modern U.S. society, where independence tends to be very highly valued.[5] Yet the physical realities of some diseases are relatively constant, and thus the line between the normal and the abnormal is not infinitely malleable.

We also must consider the nonphysical impact of this type of genetic manipulation on the women whose bodies would be its likely locus. Some of the concerns advanced in previous chapters seem to raise red flags here — for instance, the danger that *any* embrace of genetic manipulation will threaten to increase the social perception of women as reproductive "machines" who produce a "product" (i.e., children). Yet although this danger certainly seems problematic as we move toward a more complete "designing" of children, it is difficult to see how the single step of genetically preventing a serious disease such as CF seriously risks this outcome. It is true that this form of genetic manipulation, like all forms, could further fragment the experiences of conception, gestation, and birth, and women might come to view themselves, and be viewed by society generally, as more akin to "breeders." This is indeed bothersome. Yet the level of rational "design" involved in the effort to prevent serious disease seems to be a great deal lower than in the positive choice of, say, a child's eye or skin color, memory ability or intelligence level, or even gender. In other words, the risk of altering the social perception of women in this way may, in *this* case, be relatively low and thus may be a risk worth taking for the sake of promoting the health and life of the child.

Finally, we must consider how this sort of genetic manipulation may affect the definition of parenthood that society holds generally. Given the normative view of human well-being presented here, the act of taking steps, even genetic steps, to relieve severe physical suffering for a future child seems very much in keeping with a view of parenthood whereby parents' primary role is to accept, love, and nurture their children. In other words, to seek to relieve the suffering of a child is a far cry from seeking perfection in that child. Although parents must, as far as they can, carefully consider the likely level of actual suffering for their particular child, it is difficult to maintain that parents who choose to help their children in this way are contradicting the nurturing, loving, accepting family environment that a feminist Christian vision promotes.

Recommendations

All things considered, genetic manipulation for the prevention of cystic fibrosis, and likely, by extension, other very serious diseases, seems in keeping with human flourishing. If it could be done well, such manipulation would relieve tremendous amounts of human suffering and greatly increase the level of human flourishing in children who otherwise would contract the disorder. Moreover, it very likely would ease the enormous burden currently borne by so many parents of children with CF, especially more severe cases of the disease. Many of the less tangible dangers associated with genetic manipulation that are presented as a part of this work — for example, the social degradation of women, or inordinately high expectations placed upon genetically manipulated children — are relatively less likely to occur with this type of genetic manipulation as compared with the other forms under consideration.

Of course, as the technology itself moves closer to the point of implementation, society must move with extreme caution on several counts. First and foremost, significant gains must be made in terms of physical safety for both mother and child; this must not become yet another realm in which women's health is jeopardized in the name of scientific "progress," or where children's overall physical well-being is compromised because of Western society's fascination with high-tech "fixes" to health problems. Furthermore, we as a society must insist that access to the technology's benefits be extended to all, regardless of ability to pay; and if possible this must be done in the context of an expanding healthcare pie, so that this sort of high-tech measure does not significantly keep us from fulfilling other, more low-tech compelling healthcare needs.

The Case of Down Syndrome

Before moving on to our second example of genetic manipulation, it is worth considering briefly whether or not a similar analysis could be applied to other, sometimes less serious genetic disorders. Trisomy 21, the indicator of what is commonly referred to as Down syndrome, is a much more common disorder with a wide variation in severity.[6] Children with milder cases of Down syndrome often grow up to hold jobs and maintain a relatively high measure of independence. At the other end of the spectrum, some people affected by the disorder experience severe mental retardation. Down syndrome can, in some cases, be considered a less severe genetic disorder than CF, though it too can take graver forms. In any case, it is statistically far more common than CF.

It is impossible adequately to evaluate the application of genetic manipulation to Down syndrome without engaging in a more thorough analysis of the disorder itself. Yet the structure of the analysis applied here is useful in evaluating this and other genetic disorders. Does Down syndrome compromise the integral well-being of children who have it? In what sense are others, especially those most closely related to such children, affected? What are the dangers associated with the development of genetic manipulation to prevent Down syndrome? What will be the emotional and relational impact on a child who learns that he or she has (or has not) been genetically manipulated with respect to this disorder? What will be the emotional and relational impact on the women who parent such children, and on women in general? Finally, what socioeconomic considerations must be taken into account in order to preserve basic socioeconomic equality, especially in terms of access to healthcare, while also identifying and preserving what might be considered a "good" social diversity?

Down syndrome may be a more complicated case for analysis because one of its main symptoms is mental retardation, a condition that is emotionally and ethically charged, particularly in a society that highly values success and achievement, perhaps to a fault. In other words, social construction of the disorder plays a more significant role here than it does with CF, which is characterized more purely by its physical symptoms. In a similar vein, there exists ongoing debate about whether persons with mental retardation actually experience significant suffering from their condition, or, alternatively, whether a fearful general population falsely attributes such suffering in order to cover up its own uneasiness with the symptoms of mental retardation. Retardation is not the same thing as suffering.[7] An adequate analysis will examine these dimensions more deeply, particularly attending to the actual well-being of those afflicted by Down syndrome and those most directly affected by genetic manipulation designed to prevent it. The key here, as in the analysis of CF, is whether Down syndrome itself, as well as genetic "treatment" for its prevention, produces a state, individually or socially, that is significantly dysfunctional — that is, one that clearly contradicts integral human flourishing. In general, extreme cases of significant suffering (if such cases can be accurately predicted) will be more likely to merit the interventions of genetic manipulation, since they more obviously contradict human well-being.

Improving on the Normal: The Case of Memory Enhancement

If genetic manipulation for the prevention of cystic fibrosis falls toward one end of the therapy enhancement spectrum, the genetic enhancement of memory falls near the other. Except in rare cases where an individual's memory is so impaired that it inhibits ordinary daily activity, most would consider memory enhancement to carry us beyond what can be considered "normal" human functioning.[8] Of course, as I have pointed out at various junctures in this book, it is impossible to evaluate what is "normal" without attending to social context and expectation. Routine childhood immunizations provide an apt example; most of us, at least in developed Western societies, have come to expect the immunities that they confer as basically "normal," though this certainly was not the case a century ago. These immunizations, in truth, represent a form of medical enhancement.

Nevertheless, the "normal" is not infinitely pliable. A working understanding of what counts as a normal memory might be reached by turning again to the basic definition of human well-being elaborated by Nussbaum. A certain ability of memory is required in order for a human being to enjoy basic well-being: to imagine, think, and reason; to have attachments to things and persons outside of oneself; to form a conception of the good and to engage in critical reflection about the planning of one's own life, and so forth. Additionally, a basic amount of memory is an essential requirement for the continuity of the "self" in an individual, as that term is ordinarily understood. It is this level of memory that we can label "normal" for purposes of analysis vis-à-vis genetic enhancement.

The case of memory is even more complicated by the close connection between memory and intelligence. Intelligence levels are not simply a matter of raw data; intelligence is far more socially constructed than we are prone to recognize. No one really knows the various factors that play into what is ordinarily labeled "intelligence," nor exactly how heredity (versus environment) plays a role. It is only recently that categories such as "emotional intelligence" have been discussed at all, and standard IQ tests have come to be recognized in many circles as inadequately reflecting the many and varied forms that intelligence can take.[9] Many scholars have also cautioned that standardized intelligence testing reflects socioeconomic biases that disadvantage poorer and/or nonwhite persons. Furthermore, different forms of intelligence will be differentially valued in dissimilar societies; in the modern United States, for instance, it happens that scientific-technical knowledge is far more valued than it was, say, one hundred years ago, or than it would be in the context of a rural, less developed economy.

Still, few would dispute that memory appears to play a strong role in what is ordinarily considered intelligence. Many among us undoubtedly would like to possess a better memory, to better be able to recall names, facts, details, or experiences from time to time, and to enjoy the mental "edge" that such a change would likely produce in our intellectual experience. The question before us at this juncture is whether or not the use of genetic manipulation to achieve such memory enhancement will ultimately serve or impede human flourishing, according to the picture of human well-being described in this book.

Examining Arguments against Genetic Manipulation

Physical Considerations

Turning first to the issue of physical safety, we find that many of the hesitations expressed in the discussion of cystic fibrosis also apply here. There are massive safety hurdles that would need to be overcome before we could even begin to consider such interventions as positively serving physical well-being. Again, it is not only the safety of the child whose genome is "designed" in this way that must be considered; it is also the safety of the women whose bodies would very likely be the locus, at least secondarily, for proactive genetic procedures (e.g., involving embryos or gametes). These safety hurdles are even more troubling in the case of memory enhancement than they are with CF, since here we lack the immediate justification that the procedure in question, though dangerous, would be designed to overcome a bodily ailment that itself may be regarded as dangerous.

Emotional and Relational Considerations

Genetic manipulation for memory enhancement may also specifically compromise women's well-being in other, less direct ways. Women have good reason to fear the increased medicalization of the reproductive process and the entrusting of their reproductive health to a still heavily male-dominated medical profession. Historically, the shift toward the medicalization of reproduction has simply not served women's overall physical, or even emotional, well-being. This shift has translated into a decrease in the locus of body control from women's perspective, with serious physical as well as psychological ramifications. In the context of a haunting history of medical abuses, women should be concerned about any further medicalization of the reproductive process, particularly when there is no "disease" to be treated or prevented. It is, of course, true that genetic manipulation may prove different from these earlier offenses, since presumably it would take place in an era of heightened awareness of women's health issues; nevertheless, it represents a further intrusion of technology into women's reproductive lives, and women have good reason to be wary of this.

Also, there is the concern that this form of genetic manipulation, like that used to prevent CF, will encourage an already all-too-common willingness on the part of some medical professionals and the general public to view woman's social role as akin to that of a breeder. In fact, it is reasonable to assert that this fear is even more well-founded in the case of genetic enhancement than with disease prevention, since here the level of rational, proactive design — that is, beyond what is considered "normal" — increases. In other words, we are now facing not just the rectification or prevention of a serious physical dysfunction, but rather a positive step toward "engineering" a particular kind of child. The distinction is subtle; indeed, no doubt some would disagree that any such distinction is warranted at all, since in both cases a parent takes steps to "design" a child in a particular way. Yet, at a minimum, it seems likely that the experience and self-perception of a pregnant woman who takes steps to prevent CF in her child will be significantly different from that of a woman who takes steps to enhance her child's memory. To perform the former is well in keeping with our ordinary understanding that a parent's role includes protecting and fostering the health and basic well-being of a child, whereas to perform the latter begins to reach beyond that understanding to a new and more directive role for parents in regard to their offspring's care: engineering beyond what is widely considered "normal" in order to meet individual specifications. It is my contention here that this new, more directive role conduces too readily to the perception of procreation as production, and thus to the corresponding perception that women function a bit like reproductive machines in the procreative process.

What of the experience of the child who is genetically enhanced in order to have an improved memory? It does seem likely that a child whose memory has been enhanced genetically will experience more pressure to perform intellectually than peers. In effect, the child will be forced to focus on memory, and perhaps more generally on cognitive abilities, in a way that otherwise might have not occurred. The child will not be able to exist in the world without reflecting about this aspect of being, knowing that the parents *chose* that he or she should excel in this way and indeed took steps to try to ensure it.[10] In fact, the nonengineered peers of such a child will be in a similar situation because they too will be forced by their circumstances to reflect on their own cognitive abilities, and particularly how they "measure up" in a world where some children's memories are enhanced, and others are not. These dynamics may not have devastating effects on the self-esteem of these children or produce debilitating identity crises, but it is not difficult to see that they compromise children's well-being in a profound, if subtle, manner.

There also exists the danger that a child whose memory has been enhanced will experience unforeseen negative side effects of a superior memory, indeed perhaps well beyond childhood. Many of us, for instance, would prefer not to remember some details of our childhood, particularly those most embarrassing or painful. Will a child (and, later, adult) whose memory has been enhanced be imprisoned by the past in unexpected ways? Will this mental "edge" prove to be more akin to a double-edged sword, allowing the person to think sharply and quickly but also tormenting him or her with information from the past (distant or immediate) that gets in the way of present-day functioning, even flourishing? These questions may be impossible to answer, but they should raise profound doubts that a genetically enhanced memory is of unequivocal benefit, from the child's point of view.

Even aside from the child's immediate experience of this sort of genetic manipulation, the techniques themselves may contribute to an inappropriate understanding of children, more than would be the case with the prevention of CF. It is easy to see how the genetic enhancement of memory — that is, genetic manipulation without the justification of preventing the suffering associated with serious disease — could begin to lead parents down a path of viewing their children as a particularly valuable form of property. Restoring a child to health, and, by extension, trying to ensure basic good health to begin with, is qualitatively different from seeking out ways to enhance or "perfect" that child's experience of the world; the latter moves away from the accepting and nurturing environment that children's flourishing requires and begins to hint at a parental perfectionism whereby parents risk overlooking, or at least dangerously downplaying, the basic well-being of the child. Such a tendency could lead to, among other things, parents with dramatically and perhaps unrealistically raised expectations for their children, expectations that, when unmet, might provoke enormous disappointment in those parents, who may have invested a great deal of money and effort to "engineer" their children's genes in the first place.

The danger is perhaps especially acute in the case of memory enhancement (or the enhancement of any other recognizable component of intelligence). It is quite easy to envision anxious parents embracing this technology in the name of furthering their child's "best interests," while their actual (even if unrecognized) goal is to have a "high-quality" child who can and will compete effectively in a highly competitive world. This is precisely the sort of distortion examined in chapter 2: the child is viewed less as an individual human being with personal needs and interests, and more as an extension of the parents and in terms of her or his quality and ability to "measure up." In other words, the child is increasingly understood to be akin to an especially treasured form of private property rather than viewed as one party in a relationship marked by mutual love and respect. I do not mean to deny that the child someday may come to appreciate having a superior memory, or even to understand such a quality as being essentially in her or his own best interests. Even if that were to happen, that belief may in fact betray the child's own self-expectation of perfect intellectual performance. In other words, a girl, say, with genetically enhanced memory may have come to believe that she is not a valuable person unless she outperforms her peers intellectually. If this is the case, she will have come to internalize the perfectionist mindset that her parents have set in motion for her life, the belief that basic worth is a function of a person's "quality" of performance (or looks, or skin color, or the like) rather than a person's status as a human being and a child of God. It seems quite likely that this kind of hypercritical self-perception could lead to the sort of free-floating anxiety and related personality disorders described in chapter 2 of this book, ultimately inhibiting the child's willingness freely to enjoy life.

A parent who participates in this sort of scenario may have begun to cross the dangerous line (even if unwittingly) whereby he or she ceases to accept and love the child unconditionally — that is, even in the face of imperfection and disappointment. Hence, rather than fostering a parenting style marked by acceptance and nurture, a society that encourages this shift will subtly advocate a perfectionist parental mindset, which focuses inordinately on the "quality" of the child. To focus this way, and not on characteristics that are central to the child's basic well-being, threatens to conditionalize parenthood to an unacceptable degree.[11] It lends itself far too easily to the public commodification of children, particularly in U.S. society, where there is a proneness to commodifying everything in public life. It runs the risk of exacerbating an already existent societal tendency of intolerance toward that which is "imperfect," potentially reducing social support for those persons who are not a part of (to use Stanley Hauerwas's image) "the Pepsi generation." Finally, the level of parental control that is represented by the effort to "perfect" a child genetically flies directly in the face of the Christian insight that a child is not properly understood as the object of ownership or practical design at all, but rather is a gift entrusted to a parent's care, meriting a parent's awe, respect, and unconditional love.

Again, the same dangers may exist to a lesser degree with disease prevention. But the prevention of disease, at least a serious disease such as cystic fibrosis, is much more obviously in keeping with our basic picture of human flourishing. A parent's attempt to prevent a child from contracting CF could possibly represent the beginnings of a perfectionist mindset, and it certainly can be considered a small step toward focusing on the "quality" of the child. Indeed, on one level, the acceptance of a child with a disability itself conveys just the sort of unconditional love and acceptance that Christianity traditionally advocates. However, the choice to genetically prevent CF may also simply represent a genuine concern to avoid unnecessary suffering in that child, suffering that directly and profoundly contradicts the child's basic well-being. Surely it is much easier to imagine that a parent making such a choice could nevertheless display a higher degree of acceptance and even unconditional love toward that child than a parent who moves to the level of genetic manipulation for memory enhancement.[12] Moreover, it seems likely that a child whose memory has been genetically enhanced will experience far more pressure to "perform" in life (in this case, intellectually) than one who has been genetically prevented from living with the symptoms of a serious disease such as cystic fibrosis. In fact, the two children's experiences of parental and social expectation probably will be entirely distinct.

Socioeconomic Considerations

What does the picture look like when we turn to the larger socioeconomic implications of memory enhancement? One of the most troublesome considerations is that memory enhancement, as it becomes increasingly common, could very well function to exacerbate and serve insidious race and class prejudices. As with other forms of genetic manipulation, it seems likely that only those with better access to the healthcare system generally will be able to take advantage of the benefits of this technology. In fact, this is even more true with memory enhancement than it is with disease prevention, since enhancement is much less likely to merit the public expenditure of scarce healthcare dollars. Hence, if the genetic enhancement of memory were to become widely adopted, no doubt we would see it being disproportionately utilized by the wealthier segments of society — people who already have significantly more means at their disposal to help their children excel academically and socioeconomically. From the point of view of poorer members of society (who, historically, are disproportionately nonwhite), this use of the technology can only further entrench the socioeconomic disparities that they already face on a daily basis.

Furthermore, one can legitimately ask whether public funds would be better spent elsewhere, on services that meet more basic healthcare and other social needs. Indeed, from a feminist and Christian point of view — that is, one that opposes dramatic socioeconomic disparities and advocates a preferential option for the poor in the name of promoting the common good — we must insist that these basic needs be more adequately addressed before we as a society even consider support for genetic enhancement. It is impossible to ignore that more funding for Head Start programs or WIC (Special Supplemental Nutrition Program for Women, Infants, and Children) will have a far more positive overall social effect than would funding for this form of genetic enhancement. Perhaps it is true that, in a capitalist economy, one cannot prevent wealthier individuals from using private means to finance the genetic enhancement of their offspring. Yet, as noted above, enormous amounts of public funds have already been devoted to research that ultimately would support these technologies, and society has a legitimate interest in specifying how their benefits are ultimately allotted. Moreover, the huge medical infrastructure necessary to develop and implement technologies of genetic manipulation inevitably drains personnel and resources away from other, perhaps more pressing, medical and public health needs.

The history of eugenics outlined in chapter 2 should give us even further pause as we evaluate genetic enhancements such as that of memory. In the past, often well-intentioned social reformers promoted eugenic practices as benefiting society generally, all the while oblivious to the ways in which such practices in fact expressed and entrenched harmful socioeconomic prejudices. The case of Carrie Buck provides only one example, albeit an excellent one, of how we as a society can so easily be blind to our own biases — in this case, allowing the involuntary sterilization of a woman who, by later accounts, suffered from little else than socioeconomic disadvantage and bad luck.[13] The relative ease with which U.S. society appears to have accepted this sort of abuse, as well as the later horrors practiced especially in Nazi Germany, should not necessarily lead us to reject all forms of genetic manipulation, but it should make us extremely wary of how these technologies can serve our insidious social prejudices.

Even apart from these unrecognized social and economic biases, the fact remains that, historically, eugenic thought, buttressed by medicine, differentially valued (and society differentially protected) persons based on their assumed intelligence, beauty, or talent, not on their basic worth as human beings. This lends credence to the fear, so often expressed by persons with disabilities, that medical genetics, in spite of its good intentions, can too easily become an instrument of oppression against those who do not fit a popular social definition of human excellence. Of course, for the reasons outlined in chapter 2, we in the West have less cause to fear today that society will forcibly impose a broad eugenic program than we do that society will move toward the embrace of a more private eugenics, one that is voluntary, and implemented individual choice by individual choice. Obvious individual abuses such as that committed against Carrie Buck may be less likely to occur under such a "democratic" and voluntary eugenics, but pernicious socioeconomic effects will remain if we are not vigilant about preventing them.

One value that works against eugenic forms of thought is the commitment to protecting a "good" diversity, as discussed earlier. Is a diversity of abilities to remember well part of such a "good" diversity? Indeed, although most people at some time in their lives wish that they could better remember things, it is not at all clear that an improved memory, and the increased cognitive abilities that such a memory confers, would be unequivocally beneficial. Perhaps, as noted before, there are benefits unknown to us of *not* being able to remember well. Moreover, perhaps society itself, and not just individuals, benefits from the collective *imperfection* of the memories of its members. Do those with inferior memories (or, by extension, intelligence levels) have something to offer society, something that would be lost if we edged toward a collectively higher intelligence (at least as measured by standard IQ tests)? Is it possible that those with inferior memories are more apt to develop other positive qualities in themselves? Christian thought, as described above, exhorts us to look hard for the good that nature presents to us, the good that may be difficult to find, initially, in "imperfection." If, for instance, persons with mental retardation have something unique to teach us about ourselves and about our communities, could the same not be true of persons with less-than-perfect memories? Let me be clear: I do not wish to suggest that conditions that result in severely impaired memories — for instance, Alzheimer's disease — positively serve human well-being. Rather, I am urging that we pause to consider the ways that imperfect memories, particularly those that nevertheless fall into the category of "normal," may actually be a part of our overall human well-being before we decide that improved memories will translate into a better society or an unequivocally better experience for individuals.

Examining Arguments for Genetic Manipulation

In spite of the foregoing arguments, there is no denying that genetically enhanced memories will likely give particular children an intellectual "edge" in school and in later life. With that edge presumably will come increased satisfaction and diminished frustration, at least for some; and these things, it must be remembered, are goods in themselves. Furthermore, it is easy to see how the improved chances of success in life that an enhanced memory could promote will be attractive to many individuals as they consider their own children's well-being. The hesitations expressed above that an amplified memory may in fact detract from well-being in some respects should not eclipse the very real desires that many individuals will have to enhance their children's well-being in these ways.

We must not hastily condemn parents for wanting to improve their children's chances for success in a competitive world. Ethicist Arthur Caplan, addressing the prospect of genetic enhancement of children, points out that parental desires to this end, though potentially problematic, are at least understandable, and they are not so very different from the urge to provide a child with private piano or tennis lessons, or high-quality nutrition. In this respect, such desires surely are understandable. He writes,

> In a world dominated by competition, parents understandably want to give their kids every advantage. There is hardly a religion on the

> planet that does not exhort its believers to enhance the welfare of their children. The most likely way for eugenics to enter our lives is through the front door as nervous parents — awash in advertising, marketing and hype — struggle to ensure that their little bundle of joy is not left behind in the genetic race.[14]

Indeed, there may in effect be very little difference between genetically enhancing a child's memory and sending that child to an expensive private school that offers a superior education. Both will have their advantages and disadvantages, and both represent a parent's efforts to make life's road smoother for the child. Both, in fact, may entail many of the pitfalls listed above — for instance, exacerbating socioeconomic stratification or raising a parent's expectations to levels that will prove unhealthy for the child. Still, one can argue that altering a child's genes is a fundamentally different endeavor from enhancing his or her education; unlike the latter, the former seeks to change the child at a biological level, about which the child has no say. The alteration of genes thus may affect the child on a deeper level, one that is more central to his or her developing sense of identity.

This is a difficult set of arguments to negotiate, but in truth we do not need to arrive at an answer in order to make a preliminary judgment about this form of genetic enhancement. Even if the genetic enhancement of memory is in fact akin to the provision of an education in certain expensive private schools, we must evaluate the genetic enhancement on its own merits and pitfalls. Indeed, the education offered in any number of high-pressure private schools may itself ultimately contradict the well-being of a child in ways not unlike the effects of genetic enhancement. The question, in either case, is whether human well-being, and in particular the well-being of the child, is promoted or hindered by the measures taken.

It may be helpful here to engage in a "thought experiment" in order to better understand the reasons someone might wish this form of genetic enhancement for their children. What if, for instance, there were a special diet available that would dramatically and safely improve one's memory? That is, what if individuals simply could choose to eat more foods that were rich in a particular vitamin that significantly aids memory? Pregnant women might even eat these foods in an effort to positively alter the memories of their (future) children. Certainly the "health" benefits of eating such foods would be touted by the food industry, and it seems perfectly understandable that many, even most, people would want to do so. Done this way, memory enhancement does not seem so menacing a prospect after all.

Of course, genetic manipulation differs from this example in a variety of ways. First, genetic manipulation is much more physically invasive than a vitamin-rich diet, and it involves, as we have seen, a great deal of physical risk. Second, the use of genetic manipulation, at least as presently envisioned, entails the medicalization of reproduction in a way that a change in diet simply would not. As I have pointed out repeatedly, women in general have much to fear from this increased medicalization and the attendant dangers that could be expected. Third, unlike the diet scenario, the development and implementation of genetic manipulation, and all of the medical infrastructure necessary to support it, is sure to be enormously expensive. These costs will be borne by all members of society, even those who do not elect to pay for the procedures themselves. Furthermore, a change in diet would be relatively easy to implement and thus relatively available to all, even those of lesser financial means, whereas genetic manipulation is sure to be disproportionately available to the wealthier members of society.

As elaborated above, however, among the most troubling aspect of the genetic manipulation of children is that it too readily conduces to the objectification of children, as well as an alteration for the worse in our generally shared understanding of the highest goals and values of parenthood. Indeed, a similar danger exists in our thought experiment: one could imagine that overzealous parents could foist a "memory diet" upon their children in much the same way, and with much the same perfectionist expectations, that they could manipulate their children genetically. In fact, neither action would unequivocally serve human (and particularly children's) well-being, although both represent quite understandable desires of parents who wish, even if anxiously, to give their children every advantage in a competitive world.

Recommendations

It is my judgment that, overall, the genetic enhancement of memory is too likely to hinder human well-being to merit our support. The increased satisfaction and diminished frustration that it could provide to individuals simply do not outweigh the many drawbacks that have been elaborated here. On balance, memory enhancement does not play the integral role in human flourishing that disease prevention does. It not only threatens the physical and, perhaps, emotional well-being of children and of women, but also it could negatively affect the larger relations that compose our society (parent-child, peer, socioeconomic, and so on), and it reflects an understanding of parenthood and of children that leads us away from our best intuitions. Hence, only when a person's memory is so severely impaired that it significantly impedes daily functioning, and thus could be considered a disease, should we contemplate supporting this form of genetic enhancement.

This conclusion should not, however, be taken to apply to all forms of genetic enhancement. Too often a bright conceptual line is drawn between therapy and enhancement that is difficult to defend when it comes to specific cases; routine childhood immunizations provide one example of a form of medical enhancement that we have widely come to accept in the name of disease prevention. Part of the point of the present work is to show that every sort of genetic manipulation must be individually examined and evaluated with respect to how it is likely to affect human flourishing, understood here to reflect feminist and Christian insights. In other words, is the procedure in question likely to aid human well-being or to obstruct it? Certain forms of enhancement can indeed harm human well-being, sometimes in ways that are not immediately obvious and therefore might be dismissed as "merely symbolic." In short, our job is to judge, to the best of our abilities, when human flourishing is well-served and when it is not.

"Shaping" Sex: The Case of Sex Preselection

The final example of genetic manipulation that I will consider here is sex preselection. This form of "designing" one's offspring is different in obvious ways from disease prevention and memory improvement, for it does not fit neatly along the traditional therapy enhancement spectrum. Furthermore, it does not, at least for now, involve the manipulation of genes already present in an embryo or gamete, but rather entails the selection of a gamete (a sperm cell) based on whether it is X- or Y-bearing, or of an embryo determined to be of the desired gender.[15] Nonetheless, in its own way, sex preselection is indeed a form of genetic manipulation, since a genetically determined characteristic of the child is effectively chosen—dictated—by the parents. Hence, many of the same considerations apply. It is also the form of genetic manipulation that is most likely to present itself as a realistic option in the near future, particularly since the development in 1999 of the MicroSort method. Indeed, the mere fact that many parents currently desire to know the gender of their children in advance (using the techniques of ultrasound and amniocentesis) attests to the likelihood, though not the certainty, that sex preselection methods eventually will develop a very real following, particularly if they become easier to implement. It is especially important, then, that we evaluate sex preselection from the point of view of broader human well-being.

Examining Arguments against Genetic Manipulation

Physical Considerations

Physically, some of the same hesitations apply here that we encountered with other forms of genetic manipulation, although the specifics are vastly different. Threats to the physical safety of the children whose sex will be preselected have not, at this point, been fully determined. The researchers who developed the MicroSort technique claim that this new method of sex selection is safer than previous ones, but the technique has not yet been implemented enough to test this claim adequately. The physical dangers to women, at least of this method, appear to be minimal, since it involves primarily artificial insemination, which has long been safely practiced and is relatively nontechnical.

Yet the picture grows murkier as we consider future developments, particularly ones that make sex preselection easier for couples to implement. One could imagine, for instance, a technique eventually being advanced whereby a woman ingests a pill or is given an injection before intercourse, affecting the likelihood that she conceives a child of one or the other gender. Such a scenario may stretch the imagination today, but if developed, it very likely would be wildly popular because it would make sex preselection possible without the distasteful step of artificial insemination. Such a technique would pose serious safety questions for the conceiving women, questions that must be thoroughly examined and put to rest if well-being is to be protected. The historical context does not inspire confidence. We thus have excellent reason to be wary, and to insist that women's (and children's) physical well-being be thoroughly taken into account in the development of any sex preselection technique, current or future.

On the other side of the physical well-being equation lies the fact that many girls who are born unwanted into the world experience immense amounts of physical suffering. This is especially true in developing countries where most families may have few resources to go around, and girl children are seen as a particular financial burden. We have already noted the overall preference worldwide for boys, and the consequent practices of selective abortion and even widespread female infanticide in some areas are at this point well-documented. Furthermore, when resources are scarce, girl children more often experience malnutrition and premature death, not to mention a lack of educational opportunities and chances for meaningful work.[16] In short, the well-being of girls is often dramatically compromised in a patriarchal world, where all too often they are seen more as burdens than blessings.

A commitment to reduce human suffering cannot ignore these realities as the context for sex preselection. It is quite likely that sex preselection techniques, if made reliable, accessible, and affordable, would be widely adopted in societies that now hold a preference for boys, and where many of these more troubling practices take place. Hence, sex preselection could in fact dramatically reduce the levels of suffering and death now faced by so many girl children. In other words, if couples were given the option of preselecting for boy children, they would less often need to make the decision of whether or not to kill or otherwise mistreat their (unwanted) daughters. Even in societies in which female infanticide is not widely practiced, it is conceivable that some parents would choose to have boys rather than girls in order to spare their children the patriarchal restrictions that girls so routinely experience.

As argued in chapter 3, however, this is a problematic "solution" at best when taken in the aggregate. The more concrete social implications of sex preselection will be discussed below; here I simply note again that the well-being of any group of people, including women and girls, is generally not well-served by the reduction or elimination of that group itself. Feminists must insist that social patterns and practices change to be more welcoming and inclusive of girls and women, long before we consider that sex preselection to reduce the number of unwanted girls (and women) presents any sort of long-term acceptable solution. Hence, even if sex preselection would reduce the occasions of sex-based suffering, feminists must reject it as an integral strategy to support women's flourishing.

Emotional and Relational Considerations

The stakes rise when we turn to emotional and relational well-being as components of human flourishing. Perhaps one of the most troubling dangers of sex preselection in this regard is that such a choice may reflect an inordinate emphasis on secondary human characteristics — that is, characteristics that are not central to human worth. In other words, adults who would go so far as to predetermine the gender of their children in fact may not be accepting those children fully, on a deep and perhaps even unrecognized level, for the valuable human beings that they are. Rather than reflecting that children are dignified individuals in their own right — a fundamental point of feminist and

Christian thought — this approach may indicate that an adult is prone to creating a child primarily in order to fulfill his or her own needs.

Of course, one can argue that most parents have children for a combination of reasons, and that it is unrealistic to demand that parents have entirely "pure" motives, free from all self-interest, when they choose to have children in the first place. Nevertheless, there is a limit to the level of considering one's own self-interests that is healthy or acceptable in the decisions of whether or not to have a child and of how to raise that child. When a child is conceived entirely in order to fulfill an unmet parental need, and raised with only the desires of the parents in mind — that is, with little or no real recognition of or respect for the particularity of the child per se — we can rightly charge that the child is being inappropriately objectified. In that case, the child is being treated more as a possession than as a person in her or his own right, deserving of awe and respect.

It is debatable, to be sure, whether or not preselecting a child's sex participates in this inappropriate level of objectification. Certainly the child whose gender has been preselected, and who knows it, will quite likely experience an increased level of pressure to be a certain way — that is, to meet the hopes and expectations of the parent (or parents) who made the choice. The level to which this parental expectation impinges on the child's freedom may, of course, prove mild. A greater danger exists that the child will grow up knowing that his or her "place" in the birth order was preselected. If the statistics are true that in the United States males are more often desired as firstborn children and females as second-born children, then we can rightly fear that a disproportionate number of boys will grow up knowing that they were chosen to be first, and likewise that a disproportionate number of girls will grow up knowing that they were selected to be second. One can imagine the deep sense of inferiority that such a dynamic could engender in younger sisters, an inferiority that may already be present simply because of the sexist social world of which they are a part. The question, then, is not simply whether or not children will feel accepted by parents for who they are; it also is whether children will feel completely welcomed into this world and into their own families as full and equal members.[17]

On the other hand, children who were preselected to be of one or the other sex could feel particularly wanted, treasured precisely *because* they are of a sex that was especially desired by their parents. It is crystal clear that sex-based preferences do exist, and that most parents at least perceive that the experiences of parenting boys and girls are likely to be quite different. It is common that couples wish to parent just girls, or just boys, or both, and it may be assumed that the chosen child of such a couple will be treated as specially valued. Of course, as described above, such parental sex preferences may have much to do with gender-related expectations that may be considered sexist — for instance, the idea that boys necessarily drift far emotionally from their parents, or that girls cannot share a passion for football with their fathers. Part of the contribution of feminist thought has been to point out that such rigid sex-role stereotyping ultimately functions to limit children (and adults) as individuals and deprives society of many valuable contributions that women and men (who do not fit neatly into these stereotypes) can make. Hence, challenging such assumptions in the process of parenting may represent a significant step toward a higher level of acceptance of and respect for children as they are, and ultimately it will contribute to a richer social environment.

To be sure, it is conceivable that couples would desire to parent a child of one or the other gender even if society were relatively free of these sex-role stereotypes. Even with the acknowledgment that such preferences exist, it is not necessarily the case that we should encourage parents to indulge their preferences. This is particularly true because current societies are *not* free of gender stereotyping, and it is impossible, or at least terribly difficult, conceptually to separate when a parent's hope for a child of one or the other gender participates in and supports sexist stereotypes from when it does not. Even in a nonsexist world, if a parent were to treasure a child particularly for being of the desired gender, the question arises as to whether that child will have a sense of self-worth inordinately tied to gender rather than simply regarding himself or herself as a fully dignified and unique individual. In other words, a child who feels treasured *because* of being a boy or girl arguably places a harmful level of emphasis on his or her own gender. To complicate matters further, in the real (and still patriarchal) world, children surely are less likely than their adult parents to have the mental wherewithal to resist sexist stereotypes; that is, they are more likely to adopt these harmful stereotypes into their own self-image. At least on the level of the child per se, sex preselection may fortify a tendency to link worth, even self-worth, to gender in an unhelpful way.

What about the effect of sex preselection on the parents and, perhaps more significantly, on our broader understanding of parenting itself? As it did with the other forms of genetic manipulation examined above, the account of human flourishing that I have envisioned here must question whether or not sex preselection will subtly alter how parents understand their own role and how we as a society understand the role of parents. I have emphasized that our best insights about parenting should lead us to expect that parents approach their task not as one of shaping and controlling their children, out of some sense of parental entitlement, but rather as one of loving, accepting, and nurturing them. Such an attitude necessarily will entail some level of risk and vulnerability, as parents are encouraged to forgo the unreasonably high levels of control to which genetic manipulation may in some cases conduce. Along these lines, journalist Bill Hall describes his view that sex preselection, by removing part of the surprise from the process of having children, may tend to torpedo valuable parental lessons:

> Most of all, you don't think as the years go by of your kids as the boy child or the girl child; you think of them as Mike or Stacy, as individual human beings, remarkable to you for far more than chromosomes. There is something enlightening about that. Life teaches us what to value far more with surprises than by letting us place specific orders. Getting exactly what we want out of life each time we ask tends to narrow a person rather than delight him.[18]

According to this view, giving in to the desire to control the gender of a child may work against the valuable recognition that children are unique and worthy in themselves, not because of their gender. In this way, sex preselection may ultimately function to diminish the ideal of parenting and to "narrow" parents themselves. Although the choice to preselect for sex does not necessarily indicate by itself that parents are trying to exercise an inappropriate level of control over their offspring, it may subtly begin to shape parents' own self-understanding away from the ideals that this feminist Christian account advocates.

Socioeconomic Considerations

Turning to the broader, social level, we are faced with still more questions. First, is there any merit to the argument that sex preselection reinforces a social tendency to link sex to worth, ultimately harming the cause of male-female social equality? Even some supporters of sex selection as a valid way of exercising procreative liberty are troubled by this prospect. Indeed, feminists are correct that to preselect for sex, in the context of a sexist society, will likely serve to strengthen popular conviction that prominent gender differentiation is somehow valid, and, at least in some cases, that gender *is* somehow connected to human worth. The choice to preselect for boys no doubt will function in the minds of many to confirm an already existent public bias that males are, on some level, superior to females. Even the choice to preselect for girls could function to augment gender stereotypes in the public mind — that is, if couples desire a daughter because girls are "cuter" or more adoring. In these ways sex preselection may function to reinforce patriarchal attitudes and practices; at a minimum, it will do little to challenge them. Thus, even when individual parents have the most benign of motives for desiring a child of one or the other sex, they may unwittingly play into a larger social story wherein gender is accorded an inappropriate level of prominence and is connected, however indirectly, to human worth.

Of course, there are many other ways — concrete and non-"symbolic" — that sex preselection, practiced broadly, may pose a threat to male-female social equality. These have already been elaborated above; here it is sufficient to summarize that, minimally, there exists the strong possibility that sex preselection could lead to harmfully high sex ratios in some parts of the world, and to disproportionate numbers of second-born girl children in North America. If social equality between men and women is considered a part of integral human flourishing, as is argued in this book, then we must insist that even this strong possibility should constitute a significant deterrent to, albeit not a final rejection of, sex preselection.[19] In other words, we cannot afford to take less than seriously the possibility that male-female relations would be harmed by sex preselection, for social equality is simply too significant an aspect of women's well-being to put at risk in the name of procreative liberty.

Will sex preselection affect socioeconomic stratification per se? Unlike the other forms of genetic manipulation considered in this book, sex preselection obviously will not conduce to a significant deepening of harmful gaps between rich and poor, at least in societies (such as U.S. society) where no marked overall preference for boys exists. In other words, it is not the case that the wealthy and middle classes, by virtue of their greater ability to afford this technology, will disproportionately enjoy some clear socioeconomic benefit.[20] On the other hand, in societies where having girl children poses a distinct economic disadvantage, it is more conceivable that the practice of sex preselection could aggravate social inequality. In such societies the existence of various strongly held social traditions — for instance, that parents of girls pay high dowries upon their marriage, or that it is adult sons who ensure the well-being of aging parents — could mean that the relatively expensive procedure of sex preselection ultimately could translate into further economic advantage for those who can afford it, since they would be able to assure themselves of male offspring. Certainly it will mean that these more financially well-off parents will have additional options open to them for sex selection beyond the methods that already exist (e.g., infanticide, or amniocentesis combined with selective abortion). On the one hand, we may applaud the fact that sex preselection could offer such new, and arguably less destructive, options to these parents. On the other hand, a feminist Christian account must again insist that, if such options are to be made available, they be made available to rich and poor alike, and that they not detract from other, more low-tech efforts to improve overall public health.

In the United States questions of economic justice vis-à-vis sex preselection have particular force when we contemplate the appropriate use of scarce medical resources. It seems, at a minimum, questionable that valuable healthcare dollars should be spent on the research and development of sex preselection techniques — techniques that, except in cases of sex-linked disease, will serve nonurgent needs — when so many people go without even the most basic forms of medical care. Again, even if private individuals choose to access sex preselection techniques at their own expense, it remains the case that such decisions do indirectly impact the overall distribution of medical personnel and services in this country.

Even apart from arguments having to do with social and economic justice, there is the final consideration that the existence of both males and females in this world must be considered a part of a "good" diversity according to feminist Christian tenets. The feminist principle of inclusivity not only challenges us to view males and females alike as valuable members of society, but also moves us to demand the full inclusion of women into all socioeconomic realms, especially those to which women have traditionally been given only limited access. For its part, the Christian story, at least as interpreted here, understands both men and women as reflecting the image of God. Both are cherished as children of God, and sex diversity itself is part of the wonder of God's creation. By either account, sex is not a disease; it is not dysfunctional; indeed, it is a treasured aspect of the human condition. It is not something to be "corrected," by genetic or any other means.

The foregoing considerations should lead us to be extremely wary of sex preselection, particularly if it grows to enjoy widespread appeal. True to the picture of human flourishing presented here, we must seek a world where the physical health of all people is protected; where women and men enjoy social equality; where we practice a socioeconomic system marked by equitable sharing and social solidarity; and where parents do not treat their children as private property, but rather learn to value, support, and nurture their children as the intrinsically worthy children of God that they are. In pursuit of such a world, sex preselection often may not be the best choice for parents, or for society, to make. Accordingly, we should approach the practice of sex preselection with extreme caution.

Examining Arguments for Genetic Manipulation

On the opposite side of the equation, to be sure, there are individual cases in which sex preselection may actually function to reduce extreme forms of human suffering and to advance human well-being. One of the most obvious of these is the case in which sex is preselected in order to avoid the inheritance of sex-linked genetic diseases such as muscular dystrophy or hemophilia. In such instances a child's gender is not itself the direct object of choice, but rather may be considered, in effect, a by-product of the choice to avoid the disease in question. In other words, the direct object of choice here is for a child who will not suffer from these diseases, not for a child who is female or male; the gender is an indirect object of choice. Any account that concerns itself with human flourishing as centrally as this one does must consider that flourishing may be well served in such an instance.

Likewise, there are cases, particularly in societies where girls today often are killed or severely maltreated, in which sex preselection appears to serve human well-being, at least in individual instances. As expressed above, however, we must stop short of advocating sex preselection on a broad scale as a remedy for this sort of social malady; rather, we must first insist that society recognize the worth of females and treat them with the dignity and respect that they deserve as children of God. If this were done, sex preselection presumably would not be perceived as necessary. Even while we resist advocating sex preselection as a strategy to avoid this sort of maltreatment, however, feminist Christians can recognize that in some instances sex preselection can function to reduce extreme human suffering, and that it may present the "least worst" option available to individual parents already facing exceeding hardship. Although we may not necessarily advocate sex preselection in such cases, we should minimally be less quick to condemn it.

Another possible exception to a strong bias against sex preselection is when it is done specifically for the purpose of family balancing. It is quite possible, even likely, that many parents would choose sex preselection not specifically to have either boys or girls only, but rather to have both. In other words, the parents would be selecting directly not for one or the other gender, but rather for family balance, and, again, only indirectly selecting for boys or girls at any given time. Here, rather than valuing the attributes that they associate with children of one or the other gender, some parents may cherish the healthy interaction of male and female children within the family structure. Hence, at least in some cases, the choice to preselect the sex of a second or third child to be different from that of earlier children may in fact constitute a choice to raise a family wherein boys and girls have the opportunity to grow up together and learn to respect each other as individuals.

Sex preselection for the purpose of family balancing presents a difficult and tricky issue. Certainly, many of the hesitations expressed above would still apply here. Physical dangers to the mother and/or child may still exist and would have to be overcome. Moreover, many parents who pursue this approach very often would still typecast their children according to gender, and the children themselves may be guided toward understanding their self-worth primarily in terms of their gender. Parents may learn to view their role primarily as one of shaping and controlling their children, to the ultimate detriment of family flourishing. Finally, unlike with sex-linked disease prevention, there is no overwhelming evidence here that sex preselection may function to avoid excessive forms of human suffering. The feminist Christian account presented here remains extremely wary of all these dangers.

In addition, there may exist subtle benefits to resisting a trend toward family balancing and instead maintaining a variety of family configurations, including families whose children are all of the same gender. For example, in families with either all boys or all girls, parents may be more likely to notice and value the unique characteristics of their individual children and less likely to dismiss them as gender-based. Michael Kahn, a clinical psychologist and professor at the University of Hartford, argues that "having children of the same gender forces parents to recognize a child's individual — rather than gender-specific — traits."[21] According to this view, the goal of treasuring children as dignified individuals may be well-served in all-boy or all-girl families. Furthermore, Dan Kindlon of Harvard University suggests that children in such families may have greater leeway to take part in activities generally reserved for one or the other gender; in an all-boy family, for instance, sons may have a greater chance to nurture a sibling or to help out in the kitchen — roles that otherwise may be reserved for daughters. Finally, Kahn suggests that even though parents may be more likely to participate in negative comparisons between children of the same sex, thus fostering low self-esteem, such children often are more likely to develop close sibling bonds based on shared interests.[22] All of these possibilities must be applauded for serving the feminist Christian ideals of individual respect, social equality, resistance to gender stereotyping, and mutuality.

On the other hand, the choice for family balancing also has distinct advantages, at least in some cases. It may, for instance, serve a "good" diversity because the family itself could model this diversity and enjoy its benefits. It is clear that a great number of contemporary parents experience a deep desire to have both girls and boys; and although some of this desire no doubt can be explained by the persistence of sex-role stereotyping, it is quite conceivable that it also may reflect a natural human desire for an intimate experience of this "good" diversity. Although we are right to hesitate about such a choice, there is no obvious way that having both girls and boys in one family strongly contradicts human flourishing, as long as such a choice can be made safely, and as long as the choice itself does not betray a deeper parental tendency to objectify or control their children, submit them to negative gender stereotypes, or overvalue the secondary characteristic of gender in any given case. A feminist Christian account concerned with human flourishing perhaps will not strongly advocate sex preselection under such circumstances, but it also has excellent reasons not to strongly oppose it.

Recommendations

In sum, it is my judgment that sex preselection should be approached with extreme caution, but also that it may be allowable in certain cases. The clearest of these is when sex preselection is used as a tool to avoid extreme forms of human suffering, such as those associated with serious sex-linked disorders. In addition, in some cases sex preselection for the purpose of family balancing may function as a tool to enhance rather than diminish human flourishing. Whether or not this is true in any given case will depend heavily on the parents' attitudes and their specific reasons for desiring the family balancing in the first place. Do they wish to promote mutual respect and positive diversity within their own family setting? Or, alternatively, do they simply want both a boy with whom the father can play basketball and a girl whom the mother can dress up in pretty clothing? In other words, from a feminist Christian perspective, sex preselection for family balancing could be used either to serve or to hinder human well-being.

It is because of cases such as these that I am reluctant to advocate a total rejection of sex preselection. As with other forms of genetic manipulation, an account concerned with human well-being must carefully evaluate the degree to which well-being is served in any given case. Nevertheless, the feminist Christian account presented here does urge extreme caution, and it calls parents to challenge themselves about their underlying motives — and to recognize the ways that they themselves, as well as their children, may be negatively affected — before undertaking the choice to preselect for sex. Furthermore, from the standpoint of distributive justice and the use of scarce medical resources, any given practice of sex preselection itself may be considered relatively more suspect if its development and implementation require a greater incremental expenditure of time, effort, or financial resources, thus draining those resources away from more pressing healthcare needs.

Freedom, Flourishing, and Guidelines for Change

The preceding conclusions represent a concrete effort to negotiate the inevitable tensions that arise as we set out to define what it means to flourish as a human being in specific contexts. Humans are complex animals; our consciousness — indeed, radical self-awareness — means that attending to our integral well-being is not always a simple or straightforward matter. In agreement with strong liberals, we can affirm that our freedom is a defining aspect of our humanness. We would be foolish to treat our freedom as if it did not play any role in our ability to flourish or to live as we should. At the same time, we are finite creatures. To focus only on our freedom or individual rights, and to fail to attend to the more concrete aspects of our integral well-being (physical, emotional, relational, and social), would be radically to misunderstand and mistreat ourselves.

The feminist and Christian account constructed here calls us to accept our role as responsible co-creators and thus approach genetic manipulation as a tool that we have been given, in our freedom, to help promote human flourishing as part of the flourishing of all creation. This means that we must discern carefully when genetic intervention serves well-being and when it works against it — sometimes in ways that are not immediately apparent if we focus exclusively or even too strongly on the exercise of individual free choice. A spirit of hopeful expectation ordains that we not shy away from the ways that genetic manipulation may be used to serve God's purposes in the world, including especially its healing power. On the other hand, a keen awareness of human finitude and sin mandate that we exercise caution as we seek to discern those purposes and act to help implement them.

In particular, our desire to control our world, even with the goal of making it a "better" place, should not eclipse our very real need to recognize the beauty that is already present in it, including the beauty that is present as part of human vulnerability. Our humanness does not mean only that we are free and empowered to help "co-create" the world; it also means that we are vulnerable, both to the vicissitudes of nature and to one another. Part of our role as human beings is learning to accept, and to see the beauty in, that vulnerability. The process of having children, as much or more than any other human reality, raises up that vulnerability. Children remind us that we are not, finally, in control, for they defy our best efforts to define who they are. They are, mysteriously, of us and yet not of us; they come to us as gifts, and they remind us daily that even the most well thought-out human plans pale in comparison to the miracle of a unique human life. Even as we seek to better the lives of our children, we do well to remind ourselves of the ways that they in fact better *our* lives merely by their presence in the world, however "imperfect" they may be.

Hence, promoting human flourishing finally means not only seeking to heal or to actively advance the values and conditions that we associate with human well-being, but also learning to recognize that human well-being itself depends upon accepting some level of human vulnerability. Again, this does not mean that we must shy away from the healing power that genetic manipulation offers; rather, it means that we must pause to consider the ways in which embracing genetic manipulation as a cure-all for human woes could finally work against our integral flourishing.

It is my judgment that genetic manipulation for the prevention of cystic fibrosis generally is a morally acceptable way of promoting human well-being; that the genetic enhancement of memory, except perhaps in very severe cases, is not; and that sex preselection lies somewhere in between, meriting our extreme caution with a bias toward discouragement. Although it has not been my project here to formulate and propose public policies for implementing these judgments, one might imagine that, at a minimum, public funding be granted or denied to the development and implementation of any given procedure according to its degree of ethical acceptability. Moreover, if we are to ensure that the benefits of genetic manipulation are shared by rich and poor alike, it seems reasonable to expect that *some* restraints be placed on the ability of private individuals to participate in such procedures, at least until those procedures can also be made more accessible to all.

On the other hand, I am reluctant to urge outright legal prohibition of any but the most questionable forms of genetic manipulation, since the law seems a rather blunt instrument to address the varied circumstances under which they might be sought. As an alternative, it seems appropriate that professional guidelines be put in place (for infertility specialists, genetic counselors, human geneticists, and other clinical practitioners of genetic manipulation, including sex preselection), and also that individuals be urged to pause and consider the many facets of the choices that they face — choices that may initially seem unproblematic — in regard to genetic manipulation. This could be accomplished in part by means of detailed public education combined with private counseling for those seeking genetic manipulation, in order to broaden public awareness beyond facile assurances of reproductive freedom. Although these suggestions represent only a preliminary effort, I hope that the analysis offered here can serve policy-making efforts both in the public arena and within the profession of fertility treatment.

These judgments are, I believe, in keeping with the feminist and Christian view of human flourishing envisioned here, a view that honors not only our human freedom, but also our concrete well-being and our place in God's creation. Moreover, they are judgments that, I believe, appeal more broadly to our best insights as human persons engaged in the common pursuit of having, raising, and caring for our children. To ignore these insights would be to violate our own reality and indeed to neglect our status as dignified, and interconnected, children of God.

Notes

1. Perri Klass, "One Child, Many Influences," *New York Times,* September 9, 1998, A25.

2. Sheryl Gay Stolberg, "Youth's Death Shaking Up Field of Gene Experiments on Humans," *New York Times,* January 27, 2000, A1; "Health Officials Plan Closer Scrutiny of Gene Therapy Trials," *New York Times,* March 8, 2000, A14.

3. Paul Gelsinger, Jesse Gelsinger's father, maintains that he and his son were not adequately informed of the risks entailed in the experiments performed on Jesse. The FDA also holds that the informed-consent procedures were not properly carried out in the study. See Stolberg, "Youth's Death," A20.

4. This argument assumes a "fixed pie" of resources in the overall healthcare budget. We as a society could, of course, choose to increase the amount we spend on promoting health generally.

5. Indeed, genetic manipulation for the prevention of CF can be said to help a child ultimately to grow into a level of autonomy that is particularly culturally valued in the United States.

6. Ethical analysis of genetic manipulation for Down syndrome has indeed become a pressing task since the announcement by Japanese and German scientists in May 2000 that they have completed the DNA sequence of chromosome 21. See Nicholas Wade, "Scientists Decode Down Syndrome Chromosome," *New York Times,* May 9, 2000, D4.

7. See Stanley Hauerwas, *Suffering Presence: Theological Reflections on Medicine, the Mentally Handicapped, and the Church* (Notre Dame, Ind.: University of Notre Dame Press, 1986).

8. Here I use the word "rare" advisedly, recognizing that severe memory impairment is not at all rare in older adults, as the relatively high incidence of Alzheimer's disease attests to. For the most part, in keeping with the subject of the present work, I refer in this section to the memory enhancement of children. Analysis of Alzheimer's disease would, I anticipate, lead to conclusions much different from those expressed here, since it clearly contradicts human well-being in ways that having a "merely" average memory does not.

9. Daniel Goleman, *Emotional Intelligence* (New York: Bantam Books, 1995). See also Howard Gardner, *Multiple Intelligences: The Theory in Practice* (New York: Basic Books, 1993). In spite of these limitations, in May 1998 scientists announced the discovery of at least one gene that is associated with high intelligence. See Nicholas Wade, "Gene Linked to High I.Q. Is Reported Found with New Technique," *New York Times,* May 14, 1998, A12.

10. One might speculate as to whether this problem could be eliminated by simply not informing children about their own genetic manipulation (or lack thereof). That is, just as children conceived using donor sperm are sometimes not informed of the circumstances of their conception, children who are genetically manipulated might be kept similarly uninformed. Although this certainly presents a complicating factor to ethical analysis, I do not find it realistic that such information could be successfully withheld from children, particularly older children, in many or even most cases.

11. It must be admitted that few parents can honestly claim to love their children unconditionally all the time. The point here is not that parents do this, or even that this is how parenthood is universally socially understood. Rather, my claim is that a vision of parenthood that centrally includes a commitment to unconditional love, respect, and nurture represents our best insights into what parenthood should look like. It is a vision that we as a society would do well to protect and foster whenever possible.

12. Here I assume that such memory enhancement would augment a child's memory beyond what is considered "normal" or basic to human well-being; I am not referring to the enhancement of an obviously impaired memory that significantly hinders human flourishing.

13. See the appendix.

14. Arthur Caplan, "What Should the Rules Be?" *Time,* January 22, 2001, 42.

15. Of course, the current most common method of "preselecting" sex entails the selective implantation of embryos of one or the other gender as part of in vitro fertilization. Here I have focused more heavily on methods that are truly prospective (i.e., preconceptive) sex selection.

16. Flore Murard, "Schooling for Girls in Developing Countries Still Lags Behind," *WIN News* 24, no. 3 (1998): 12; A. R. Sarin, "Women: Half the World — Half the Power," *Journal of Obstetrics, Gynaecology and Family Welfare* 3, no. 14 (1997): 5–11; S. Ghosh, "Integrated Health of the Girl Child," *Social Change: Issues and Perspectives* 25, nos. 2–3 (1995): 44–54; S. P. Punalekar, "Culture, Political Economy and Gender Marginalisation," *Social Change: Issues and Perspectives* 25, nos. 2–3 (1995): 55–69. This is, of course, true in the United States as well, albeit to a much lesser degree. Girls in the United States generally are not the targets of sex-based infanticide, but girls and women are more likely to be poor than are boys and men, and they are routinely the targets of other sex-based forms of violence, such as domestic abuse, incest, and rape. Furthermore, women are less likely than men to be paid well for their work, and historically they have had inferior access to socioeconomic resources. See Lorna McBarnette, "Women and Poverty: The Effects on Reproductive Status," in *Too Little, Too Late: Dealing with the Health Needs of Women in Poverty,* ed. Cesar A. Perales and Lauren S. Young (New York: Harrington, 1988), 55–81.

17. This dynamic carries potential harm not just for girls; it might also negatively affect boys who, being chosen more often to be firstborn, could experience a high level of pressure to perform up to parental expectations and an artificial sense of superiority over their later siblings.

18. Bill Hall, "Selecting Baby's Sex Subverts Nature's Surprise," *Tacoma News Tribune,* September 19, 1998, A11.

19. It sometimes is suggested that if sex preselection were to begin to skew the male-female sex ratio too dramatically, legal remedies could be put in place whereby sex preselection clinics would be required to preselect one girl for every boy, or vice-versa. This approach would, of course, lessen the problem of a skewed male-female ratio (where it exists), if it could effectively be enforced. However, since the problem in the United States is more likely to be one of birth order, not of a skewed aggregate sex ratio itself, this approach may have less value here than initially appears to be the case.

20. There does exist one possible way in which widespread sex preselection could aggravate social inequality in the United States. Because firstborn children do tend to achieve greater power and prestige than do children born later in the birth order, a greater proportion of firstborn male children might translate into less social and economic power for women as a whole.

21. Quoted in Margaret Renkl, "All Boys, All Girls: The Joys and Challenges of Raising Same-Sex Siblings," *Parents,* November 2000, 216.

22. Ibid., 216–17.

Appendix

The Case of Carrie Buck

THE MOVEMENT FOR eugenic sterilization in the United States perhaps reached its moral pinnacle in 1927 with the U.S. Supreme Court case of *Buck v. Bell.* In this case Oliver Wendell Holmes, one of the most renowned jurists in U.S. history, wrote a majority opinion that upheld involuntary sterilization for a "feeble-minded" young woman, Carrie Buck. This episode in U.S. legal history not only serves as a case study in all that was wrong with eugenic sterilization policy, but also reveals some of the hidden motivations and prejudices that drove eugenic thought generally.

Carrie Buck was seventeen when she was committed to Virginia's State Colony for Epileptics and Feeble-Minded. Carrie, who was determined to have a mental age of nine years, was considered a "moron" by the standards of the day, as was her mother, Emma, who also lived at the Colony. Shortly before entering the Colony, Carrie gave birth to a daughter, Vivian, conceived out of wedlock. Soon after her commitment, the Colony's board of directors ordered Carrie to be sterilized, and a court-appointed guardian began legal proceedings on Carrie's behalf to challenge the order.

In the course of trial preparation, Harry Laughlin, of the Eugenics Record Office, was consulted for an evaluation of Carrie and Emma Buck. After studying their pedigrees and scores on the then-nascent Stanford-Binet IQ test, and without ever meeting either woman in person, Laughlin offered his "expert" opinion, in a deposition to the court, that Carrie's so-called "feeble-mindedness" was indeed hereditary: "In the case given, the evidence points strongly toward the feeble-mindedness and moral delinquency of Carrie Buck being due, primarily, to inheritance and not to environment." Laughlin's own prejudices emerge in the accompanying view he expressed that Carrie and her mother "belong[ed] to the shiftless, ignorant, and worthless class of anti-social whites of the South."[1]

What of Carrie's daughter, Vivian? Because the argument for Carrie's sterilization rested on the heritability of her "feeble-mindedness," it was crucial to the court that the child's lack of mental competency be established. Hence, a Red Cross social worker was sent to examine and evaluate Vivian, then a mere seven months old. This social worker rendered her judgment that there was something about Vivian Buck — "a look about [her] that is not quite normal." She then urged that Carrie be sterilized, opining, "I think it would at least prevent the propagation of her kind."[2] This testimony, combined with an evaluation from a Eugenic Record Office field worker that young Vivian was of below average intelligence for a child of her tender age, convinced the court that Carrie Buck's "feeble-mindedness" was indeed hereditary and that she should be sterilized against her will.

Many of the assumptions of eugenic thought are glaringly apparent in the majority opinion drafted by Holmes. Not only does he see sterilization of the "unfit" as deeply connected to the promotion of social welfare, but also he views it as part of a patriotic duty on the part of those to be sterilized:

> We have seen more than once that the public welfare may call upon the best citizens for their lives. It would be strange if it could not call upon those who already sap the strength of the state for these lesser sacrifices . . . in order to prevent our being swamped with incompetence. It is better for all the world, if instead of waiting to execute degenerate offspring for crime, or to let them starve for their imbecility, society can prevent those who are manifestly unfit from continuing their kind.

Holmes completes the thought with chilling words, now infamous: "Three generations of imbeciles are enough."[3]

Buck v. Bell represented a major victory for eugenicists and a benchmark in American law vis-à-vis involuntary sterilization. It is noteworthy that faulty science propagated by the Eugenics Record Office and the use of the early Stanford-Binet IQ test — now discredited as a test for general intelligence — were in large part responsible for Carrie Buck's sterilization. But there is also a subtext to *Buck v. Bell* that has emerged only relatively recently and that sheds significant light on what else was going on in the case of Carrie Buck.

Steven Jay Gould, a paleontologist and evolutionary biologist, has researched and written about the case of Carrie Buck, and his work casts deep doubt upon the assumptions and the motives of those who obtained Buck's sterilization order. According to Gould's research, the social worker who testified as to Vivian Buck's mental capacity also revealed that Carrie Buck was initially committed to the institution *because of her pregnancy* — that is, because she was carrying an illegitimate child (Vivian). Moreover, it appears that Carrie, who grew up in a foster home, was raped by a relative of her foster parents, resulting in that pregnancy. Gould asserts,

> Her case never was about mental deficiency; Carrie Buck was persecuted for supposed sexual immorality and social deviance. The annals of her trial and hearing reek with the contempt of the well-off and well-bred for poor people of "loose morals."[4]

Indeed, accounts of Carrie Buck as an older woman seem to support the assessment that her supposed "imbecility" was a wrong designation. In 1979 Dr. K. Ray Nelson, director of the Lynchburg Hospital, where Carrie Buck had been sterilized, located her near Charlottesville. Subsequently she was visited by Paul Lombardo of the University of Virginia, who reported thus:

> As for Carrie, when I met her she was reading newspapers daily and joining a more literate friend to assist at regular bouts with the crossword puzzles. She was not a sophisticated woman, and lacked

> social graces, but mental health professionals who examined her in later life confirmed my impressions that she was neither mentally ill nor retarded.[5]

Lombardo also tracked down the school records of Vivian Buck, before she died at the age of eight. It seems that this child, evaluated as "feebleminded" at the age of seven months, performed quite adequately in her academic subjects and was considered by her teachers to be very bright. In fact, in the spring of 1931, when she was seven years old, Vivian was on her school's honor roll.[6]

If Lombardo is to be believed, it seems clear that the case of *Buck v. Bell* reveals more about the social prejudices that infected U.S. eugenic thought than it does about a perceived danger of mental deficiency. At least in Carrie Buck's case, the victims of that prejudice were the poor, the social deviants, the misfits. Under the guise of promoting the good of the population as a whole, the rights of individuals — in particular, poor or otherwise socially deviant individuals — were trampled upon. Furthermore, values that were held generally by white, middle-class professionals were expounded at the expense of the dignity and integrity of those who, by their actions or even their very existence, seemed to challenge those values. Perhaps most significantly, the case of Carrie Buck reveals how eugenic thought differentially valued persons based on assumptions about their intelligence and talent rather than on their simple worth as human beings.

Notes

1. Steven Jay Gould, "Carrie Buck's Daughter," in *Contemporary Issues in Bioethics*, ed. Tom L. Beauchamp and LeRoy Walters (Belmont, Calif.: Wadsworth, 1994), 611; J. David Smith and K. Ray Nelson, *The Sterilization of Carrie Buck* (Far Hills, N.J.: New Horizon Press, 1989), 171.
2. Gould, "Carrie Buck's Daughter," 612.
3. United States Supreme Court, "Buck v. Bell," in Beauchamp and Walters, eds., *Contemporary Issues in Bioethics*, 608.
4. Gould, "Carrie Buck's Daughter," 612.

5. Ibid. This impression is confirmed by the accounts of several persons who knew Carrie later in life. See Smith and Nelson, *Sterilization of Carrie Buck*, esp. 214, 221.

6. Gould, "Carrie Buck's Daughter," 613; Daniel J. Kevles, *In the Name of Eugenics: Genetics and the Uses of Human Heredity* (Cambridge, Mass.: Harvard University Press, 1995), 112; Smith and Nelson, *Sterilization of Carrie Buck*, 171.

Bibliography

Anderson, French. "Human Gene Therapy." *Science* 256, no. 5058 (1992): 808–13.

———. "Human Gene Therapy: Why Draw a Line?" *Journal of Medicine and Philosophy* 14, no. 6 (1989): 681–93.

———. "The Best of Times, the Worst of Times." *Science* 288, no. 5466 (2000): 627–29.

Andolsen, Barbara Hilkert. "Agape in Feminist Theological Ethics." In *Feminist Theological Ethics: A Reader,* ed. Lois K. Daly, 146–59. Louisville: Westminster John Knox, 1994.

Annas, George J., and Sherman Elias, eds. *Gene Mapping: Using Law and Ethics as Guides.* New York: Oxford University Press, 1992.

Asch, Adrienne. "Reproductive Technology and Disability." In *Reproductive Laws for the 1990s,* ed. Sherill Cohen and Nadine Taub, 69–124. Clifton, N.J.: Humana Press, 1989.

Belkin, Lisa. "Getting the Girl." *New York Times Magazine,* July 25, 1999, 26–31, 38, 54–55.

Cahill, Lisa Sowle. "Genetics, Ethics and Social Policy: The State of the Question." In *The Ethics of Genetic Engineering,* ed. Maureen Junker-Kenny and Lisa Sowle Cahill, vii–xiii. London: SCM Press, 1998.

———. *Sex, Gender, and Christian Ethics.* Cambridge: Cambridge University Press, 1996.

Campbell, Courtney S. "Prophecy and Policy." *Hastings Center Report* 27, no. 5 (1997): 15–17.

Caplan, Arthur L. "If Gene Therapy Is the Cure, What Is the Disease?" In *Gene Mapping: Using Law and Ethics as Guides,* ed. George J. Annas and Sherman Elias, 128–41. New York: Oxford University Press, 1992.

———. "What Should the Rules Be?" *Time,* January 22, 2001, 42.

Cassidy, Joseph D., and Edmund D. Pellegrino. "A Catholic Perspective on Human Gene Therapy." *International Journal of Bioethics* 4, no. 1 (1993): 11–18.

"Census of India 2001: Provisional Population Totals." Accessed at www.cyberjournalist.org.in/census/.

Chan, C. K. "Eugenics on the Rise: A Report from Singapore." In *Ethics, Reproduction and Genetic Control,* ed. Ruth F. Chadwick, 164–71. New York: Routledge, 1992.

Cole-Turner, Ronald. *The New Genesis: Theology and the Genetic Revolution.* Louisville: Westminster John Knox, 1993.

———. "Is Genetic Engineering Co-Creation?" *Theology Today* 44 (October 1987): 338–49.

Cole-Turner, Ronald, and Brent Waters. *Pastoral Genetics: Theology and Care at the Beginning of Life.* Cleveland: Pilgrim Press, 1996.

Corea, Gena. *The Mother Machine: Reproductive Technologies from Artificial Insemination to Artificial Wombs.* New York: Harper & Row, 1985.

Cowan, Ruth Schwartz. "Genetic Technology and Reproductive Choice: An Ethics for Autonomy." In *The Code of Codes: Scientific and Social Issues in the Human Genome Project,* ed. Daniel J. Kevles and Leroy Hood, 244–63. Cambridge, Mass.: Harvard University Press, 1992.

Cystic Fibrosis Foundation. "Gene Therapy and CF." Accessed at www.cff.org.

———. "Lung Transplantation." Bethesda, Md.: Cystic Fibrosis Foundation, 1999.

———. "Progress in CF Research." Accessed at www.cff.org.

———. "What Is CF?" Accessed at www.cff.org.

Davis, Dena S. "Genetic Dilemmas and the Child's Right to an Open Future." *Rutgers Law Journal* 28, no. 3 (1997): 549–92.

Davis, Nancy Ann. "Reproductive Technologies and Our Attitudes Towards Children." *Logos* 9 (1988): 51–77.

Diprose, Rosalyn. *The Bodies of Women: Ethics, Embodiment and Sexual Difference.* London and New York: Routledge, 1994.

Duster, Troy. *Backdoor to Eugenics.* New York: Routledge, 1990.

Egozcue, J. "Sex Selection: Why Not?" *Human Reproduction* 8, no. 11 (1993): 1777.

Ehrenreich, Barbara, and Deirdre English. *For Her Own Good: 150 Years of the Experts' Advice to Women.* New York: Doubleday, 1978.

Elkind, David. *The Hurried Child.* Menlo Park, Calif.: Addison-Wesley, 1981.

Ethics Committee of the American Society of Reproductive Medicine. "Sex Selection and Preimplantation Genetic Diagnosis." *Fertility and Sterility* 72, no. 4 (1999): 595–98.

Farley, Margaret A. "Feminism and Universal Morality." In *Prospects for a Common Morality,* ed. Gene Outka and John P. Reeder Jr., 170–90. Princeton, N.J.: Princeton University Press, 1993.

———. "Feminist Ethics." In *The Westminster Dictionary of Christian Ethics,* ed. James F. Childress and John Macquarrie, 229–31. Philadelphia: Westminster, 1986.

———. "Feminist Theology and Bioethics." In *Women's Consciousness, Women's Conscience,* ed. Barbara Hilkert Andolsen, Christine E. Gudorf, and Mary D. Pellauer, 285–305. San Francisco: Harper & Row, 1985.

———. "New Patterns of Relationship: Beginnings of a Moral Revolution." *Theological Studies* 36 (1975): 627–46.

———. *Personal Commitments: Beginning, Keeping, Changing.* San Francisco: Harper & Row, 1986.

———. "Selecting Your Baby's Sex: Beware of Social Abuses." *New York Daily News,* October 11, 1998, 59.

Fletcher, Joseph. "Ethical Aspects of Genetic Controls: Designed Genetic Changes in Man." *New England Journal of Medicine* 285, no. 14 (1971): 776–83.

———. *The Ethics of Genetic Control: Ending Reproductive Roulette.* Garden City, N.Y.: Anchor Books, 1974.

———. "Indicators of Humanhood: A Tentative Profile of Man." *Hastings Center Report* 2, no. 5 (1972): 1–4.

———. "Four Indicators of Humanhood — The Enquiry Matures." *Hastings Center Report* 4, no. 6 (1974): 4–7.

Frenkiel, Nora. "'Family Planning': Baby Boy or Girl?" *New York Times,* November 11, 1993, C1, C6.

Fugger, E. F., et al. "Births of Normal Daughters After MicroSort Sperm Separation and Intrauterine Insemination, In-Vitro Fertilization, or Intracytoplasmic Sperm Injection." *Human Reproduction* 13, no. 9 (1998): 2367–70.

Galton, Francis. *Hereditary Genius: An Inquiry into Its Laws and Consequences.* Rev. ed. New York: Appleton, 1891.

———. *Inquiries into Human Faculty and Its Development.* New York: Macmillan, 1883.

Gardner, Howard. *Multiple Intelligences: The Theory in Practice.* New York: Basic Books, 1993.

Gelehrter, Thomas D., and Francis S. Collins. *Principles of Medical Genetics.* Baltimore: Williams & Wilkins, 1990.

Ghosh, S. "Integrated Health of the Girl Child." *Social Change: Issues and Perspectives* 25, nos. 2–3 (1995): 44–54.

Goleman, Daniel. *Emotional Intelligence.* New York: Bantam Books, 1995.

Gould, Steven Jay. "Carrie Buck's Daughter." In *Contemporary Issues in Bioethics,* ed. Tom L. Beauchamp and LeRoy Walters, 609–13. Belmont, Calif.: Wadsworth, 1994.

Gudorf, Christine E. "Parenting, Mutual Love, and Sacrifice." In *Women's Consciousness, Women's Conscience,* ed. Barbara Hilkert Andolsen, Christine E. Gudorf, and Mary D. Pellauer, 175–91. San Francisco: Harper & Row, 1985.

Gustafson, James M. *Ethics from a Theocentric Perspective.* Vol. 2, *Ethics and Theology.* Chicago: University of Chicago Press, 1984.

———. "Genetic Therapy: Ethical and Religious Reflections." *Journal of Contemporary Health Law and Policy* 8 (Spring 1992): 183–200.

Guttentag, Marcia, and Paul F. Secord. *Too Many Women? The Sex Ratio Question.* Beverly Hills, Calif.: Sage Publications, 1983.

Hall, Bill. "Selecting Baby's Sex Subverts Nature's Surprise." *Tacoma News Tribune,* September 19, 1998, A11.

Haller, Mark H. *Eugenics: Hereditarian Attitudes in American Thought.* New Brunswick, N.J.: Rutgers University Press, 1963.

Harkness, Georgia. *John Calvin: The Man and His Ethics.* New York: Abingdon, 1931.

Harrison, Beverly Wildung. *Making the Connections: Essays in Feminist Social Ethics.* Boston: Beacon Press, 1985.

———. *Our Right to Choose: Toward a New Ethic of Abortion.* Boston: Beacon Press, 1983.

Hauerwas, Stanley. *A Community of Character: Toward a Constructive Christian Social Ethic.* Notre Dame, Ind.: University of Notre Dame Press, 1981.

———. *Suffering Presence: Theological Reflections on Medicine, the Mentally Handicapped, and the Church.* Notre Dame, Ind.: University of Notre Dame Press, 1986.

———. *Truthfulness and Tragedy: Further Investigations into Christian Ethics.* Notre Dame, Ind.: University of Notre Dame Press, 1977.

"Health Officials Plan Closer Scrutiny of Gene Therapy Trials." *New York Times,* March 8, 2000, A14.

Holland, Suzanne, and Karen Peterson. "The Health Care *Titanic:* Women and Children First?" *Second Opinion* 18, no. 3 (1993): 10–29.

Huxley, Aldous. *Brave New World.* New York and London: Harper, 1946.

Jacobs, Paul, and Peter G. Gosselin. "An Unfolding Gene Map at 'Finish Line.'" *Los Angeles Times,* May 7, 2000, A1, A10.

Jaggar, Alison M. *Feminist Politics and Human Nature.* Totowa, N.J.: Rowman & Littlefield, 1983.

Jaroff, Leon. "Battler for Gene Therapy." *Time,* January 17, 1994, 56–57.

———. "Fixing the Genes." *Time,* January 11, 1999, 68–73.

John Paul II. "The Ethics of Genetic Manipulation." *Origins* 13, no. 23 (1983): 385, 387–89.

Johnson, Elizabeth A. *She Who Is: The Mystery of God in Feminist Theological Discourse.* New York: Crossroad, 1992.

Jones, Serene. *Feminist Theory and Christian Theology: Cartographies of Grace.* Minneapolis: Fortress, 2000.

Kass, Leon R. *Toward a More Natural Science: Biology and Human Affairs.* New York: Free Press, 1985.

Keenan, James F. "Genetic Research and the Elusive Body." In *Embodiment, Morality, and Medicine,* ed. Lisa Sowle Cahill and Margaret A. Farley, 59–73. Dordrecht, Netherlands: Kluwer Academic Publishers, 1995.

Kelly, David F. "Karl Rahner and Genetic Engineering: The Use of Theological Principles in Moral Analysis." *Philosophy and Theology* 9, nos. 1–2 (1995): 177–200.

Kevles, Daniel J. "Eugenics: Historical Aspects." In *Encyclopedia of Bioethics,* ed. Warren Thomas Reich, rev. ed., 765–70. New York: Simon & Schuster Macmillan, 1995.

———. *In the Name of Eugenics: Genetics and the Uses of Human Heredity.* Cambridge, Mass.: Harvard University Press, 1995.

King, Patricia A. "The Past as Prologue: Race, Class, and Gene Discrimination." In *Gene Mapping: Using Law and Ethics as Guides,* ed. George J. Annas and Sherman Elias, 94–111. New York: Oxford University Press, 1992.

Kitcher, Philip. *The Lives to Come: The Genetic Revolution and Human Possibilities.* New York: Simon & Schuster, 1996.

Klass, Perri. "One Child, Many Influences." *New York Times,* September 9, 1998, A25.

Kolata, Gina. "Researchers Report Success in Method to Pick Baby's Sex." *New York Times,* September 9, 1998, A1, A20.

Kühl, Stefan. *The Nazi Connection: Eugenics, American Racism, and German National Socialism.* New York and Oxford: Oxford University Press, 1994.

Landler, Mark. "Clinic Caters to Couples Seeking 'Precious Gem.'" *New York Times,* July 1, 2000, A4.

Lappé, Marc. "Eugenics: Ethical Issues." In *Encyclopedia of Bioethics,* ed. Warren Thomas Reich, rev. ed., 770–76. New York: Simon & Schuster Macmillan, 1995.

Larson, Edward J. *Sex, Race, and Science: Eugenics in the Deep South.* Baltimore: Johns Hopkins University Press, 1995.

Lebacqz, Karen, ed. *Genetics, Ethics and Parenthood.* New York: Pilgrim Press, 1983.

Lemonick, Michael D., and Dick Thompson. "Racing to Map Our DNA." *Time,* January 11, 1999, 44–51.

Lewis, C. S. *The Abolition of Man.* New York: Touchstone, 1944.

Lifton, Robert Jay. *The Nazi Doctors: Medical Killing and the Psychology of Genocide.* New York: Basic Books, 1986.

———. "Sterilization and the Nazi Biomedical Vision." In *Contemporary Issues in Bioethics,* ed. Tom L. Beauchamp and LeRoy Walters, 614–21. Belmont, Calif.: Wadsworth, 1994.

Luther, Martin. "The Estate of Marriage." In *Luther's Works,* vol. 45, ed. Walther I. Brandt, 11–49. Philadelphia: Fortress, 1962.

———. "A Sermon on the Estate of Marriage." In *Luther's Works,* vol. 44, ed. James Atkinson, 3–14. Philadelphia: Fortress, 1966.

Marteau, T. M. "Sex Selection: 'The Rights of Man' or the Thin Edge of a Eugenic Wedge?" *BMJ* 306, no. 6894 (1993): 1704–5.

McBarnette, Lorna. "Women and Poverty: The Effects on Reproductive Status." In *Too Little, Too Late: Dealing with the Health Needs of Women in Poverty,* ed. Cesar A. Perales and Lauren S. Young, 55–81. New York: Harrington, 1988.

McCormick, Richard A., S.J. "Blastomere Separation: Some Concerns." *Hastings Center Report* 24, no. 2 (1994): 14–16.

———. "Genetic Technology and Our Common Future." In *The Critical Calling: Reflections on Moral Dilemmas Since Vatican II,* 261–72. Washington, D.C.: Georgetown University Press, 1989.

———. "Therapy or Tampering: The Ethics of Reproductive Technology and the Development of Doctrine." In *The Critical Calling: Reflections on Moral Dilemmas Since Vatican II,* 329–52. Washington, D.C.: Georgetown University Press, 1989.

McGee, Glenn. *The Perfect Baby: A Pragmatic Approach to Genetics.* Lanham, Md.: Rowman & Littlefield, 1997.

McKusick, Victor A. *Mendelian Inheritance in Man: Catalog of Human Genes and Genetic Disorders.* 12th ed. 3 vols. Baltimore: Johns Hopkins University Press, 1998.

Meilaender, Gilbert. *Bioethics: A Primer for Christians.* Grand Rapids: Eerdmans, 1996.

———. "Mastering our Gen(i)es: When Do We Say No?" *Christian Century,* October 3, 1990, 872–75.

———. *Body, Soul, and Bioethics.* Notre Dame, Ind.: University of Notre Dame Press, 1995.

Mensh, Elaine, and Harry Mensh. *The IQ Mythology: Class, Race, Gender, and Inequality.* Carbondale and Edwardsville, Ill.: Southern Illinois University Press, 1991.

Midgley, Mary, and Judith Hughes. *Women's Choices: Philosophical Problems Facing Feminism.* London: Weidenfeld & Nicolson, 1983.

Minden, Shelley. "Patriarchal Designs: The Genetic Engineering of Human Embryos." In *Made to Order: The Myth of Reproductive and Genetic Progress,* ed. Patricia Spallone and Deborah Lynn Steinberg, 102–9. New York: Pergamon Press, 1987.

Murard, Flore. "Schooling for Girls in Developing Countries Still Lags Behind." *WIN News* 24, no. 3 (1998): 12.

Murray, Thomas H. *The Worth of a Child.* Berkeley: University of California Press, 1996.

National Council of the Churches of Christ/USA, Panel on Bioethical Concerns. *Genetic Engineering: Social and Ethical Consequences.* New York: Pilgrim Press, 1984.

National Human Genome Research Institute. "International Consortium Completes Human Genome Project." Accessed at www.genome.gov/11006929.

National Reference Center for Bioethics Literature. "The Human Genome Project." *Scope Note* 17. Washington, D.C.: Kennedy Institute of Ethics, Georgetown University, 1999.

Nelkin, Dorothy, and M. Susan Lindee. *The DNA Mystique: The Gene as Cultural Icon.* New York: Freeman, 1995.

Nussbaum, Martha C. "Human Capabilities, Female Human Beings." In *Women, Culture and Development: A Study of Human Capabilities,* ed. Martha Nussbaum and Jonathan Glover, 61–104. New York: Oxford University Press, 1995.

O'Donovan, Oliver. *Begotten or Made?* Oxford: Clarendon, 1984.

Office of Technology Assessment, Congress of the United States. *Human Gene Therapy: Background Paper.* Washington, D.C.: Office of Technology Assessment, 1984.

Overall, Christine. *Ethics and Human Reproduction: A Feminist Analysis.* Boston: Allen & Unwin, 1987.

Parens, Erik. "Is Better Always Good? The Enhancement Project." *Hastings Center Report* 28, no. 1, special supplement (1998): S1–S17.

Parsons, Susan Frank. *Feminism and Christian Ethics.* Cambridge: Cambridge University Press, 1996.

Paul, Diane B. *Controlling Human Heredity: 1865 to the Present.* Atlantic Highlands, N.J.: Humanities Press, 1995.

———. "Eugenic Anxieties, Social Realities, and Political Choices." In *Are Genes Us? The Social Consequences of the New Genetics,* ed. Carl F. Cranor, 142–54. New Brunswick, N.J.: Rutgers University Press, 1994.

Peters, Ted. "Designer Children: The Market World of Reproductive Choice." *Christian Century,* December 14, 1994, 1193–96.

———. *For the Love of Children: Genetic Technology and the Future of the Family.* Louisville: Westminster John Knox, 1996.

———. " 'Playing God' and Germline Intervention." *Journal of Medicine and Philosophy* 20 (1995): 365–86.

———. *Playing God? Genetic Determinism and Human Freedom.* New York: Routledge, 1997.

———, ed. *Genetics: Issues of Social Justice.* Cleveland: Pilgrim Press, 1998.

Pickens, Donald K. *Eugenics and the Progressives.* Nashville: Vanderbilt University Press, 1968.

Pier, G. B., et al. "Salmonella Typhi Uses CFTR to Enter Intestinal Epithelial Cells." *Nature* 393 (1998): 79–82.

Pollack, Andrew. "Double Helix with a Twist." *New York Times,* February 13, 2001, C1, C4.

Powledge, Tabitha M. "Unnatural Selection: On Choosing Children's Sex." In *The Custom-Made Child? Women-Centered Perspectives,* ed. Helen B. Holmes, Betty B. Hoskins, and Michael Gross, 193–99. Clifton, N.J.: Humana Press, 1981.

President's Commission for the Study of Ethical Problems in Medicine and Biomedical and Behavioral Research. *Splicing Life: A Report on the Social and Ethical Issues of Genetic Engineering with Human Beings.* Washington, D.C.: U.S. Government Printing Office, 1982.

Proctor, Robert N. "Genomics and Eugenics: How Fair Is the Comparison?" In *Gene Mapping: Using Law and Ethics as Guides,* ed. George J. Annas and Sherman Elias, 57–93. New York: Oxford University Press, 1992.

———. *Racial Hygiene: Medicine Under the Nazis.* Cambridge, Mass.: Harvard University Press, 1988.

Punalekar, S. P. "Culture, Political Economy and Gender Marginalisation." *Social Change: Issues and Perspectives* 25, nos. 2–3 (1995): 55–69.

Rahner, Karl. "The Dignity and Freedom of Man." In *Theological Investigations,* vol. 2, *Man in the Church,* trans. K.-H. Kruger, 235–63. Baltimore: Helicon, 1963.

———. "The Experiment with Man." In *Theological Investigations,* vol. 9, *Writings of 1965–1967, I,* trans. D. Bourke, 205–24. New York: Herder & Herder, 1972.

———. *Foundations of Christian Faith: An Introduction to the Idea of Christianity.* Trans. William V. Dych. New York: Crossroad, 1994.

———. "The Problem of Genetic Manipulation." In *Theological Investigations,* vol. 9, *Writings of 1965–1967, I,* trans. D. Bourke, 225–52. New York: Herder & Herder, 1972.

———. "Theology of Freedom." In *Theological Investigations,* vol. 6, *Concerning Vatican Council II,* trans. K.-H. Kruger and B. Kruger, 178–96. New York: Seabury Press, 1974.

Ramsey, Paul. *Fabricated Man: The Ethics of Genetic Control.* New Haven: Yale University Press, 1970.

———. "Manufacturing Our Offspring: Weighing the Risks." *Hastings Center Report* 8, no. 5 (1978): 7–9.

Reilly, Philip R. "Eugenic Sterilization in the United States." In *Contemporary Issues in Bioethics,* ed. Tom L. Beauchamp and LeRoy Walters, 597–606. Belmont, Calif.: Wadsworth, 1994.

———. *The Surgical Solution: A History of Involuntary Sterilization in the United States.* Baltimore: Johns Hopkins University Press, 1991.

Renkl, Margaret. "All Boys, All Girls: The Joys and Challenges of Raising Same-Sex Siblings." *Parents* (November 2000): 215–21.

Roberts, Dorothy. "Norplant's Threat to Civil Liberties and Racial Justice." *New Jersey Law Journal* 134, no. 13 (1993): 20.

Robertson, John A. *Children of Choice: Freedom and the New Reproductive Technologies.* Princeton, N.J.: Princeton University Press, 1994.

———. "Embryos, Families, and Procreative Liberty: The Legal Structure of the New Reproduction." *Southern California Law Review* 59 (1986): 943–1041.

———. "Genetic Selection of Offspring Characteristics." *Boston University Law Review* 76, no. 3 (1996): 421–82.

———. "In Vitro Conception and Harm to the Unborn." *Hastings Center Report* 8, no. 5 (1978): 13–14.

———. "Liberty, Identity, and Human Cloning." *Texas Law Review* 76, no. 6 (May 1998): 1371–1456.

———. "Procreative Liberty and the Control of Conception, Pregnancy, and Childbirth." *Virginia Law Review* 69, no. 3 (1983): 405–64.

———. "Procreative Liberty and the State's Burden of Proof in Regulating Noncoital Reproduction." *Law, Medicine, and Health Care* 16, nos. 1–2 (1988): 18–26.

Rothman, Barbara Katz. "The Meanings of Choice in Reproductive Technology." In *Test Tube Women: What Future for Motherhood?* ed. Rita Arditti, Renate Duelli Klein, and Shelley Minden, 23–33. Boston: Pandora Press, 1984.

———. "Not All That Glitters Is Gold." *Hastings Center Report* 22, no. 4, special supplement, "Genetic Grammar" (1992): S11–S15.

———. "Of Maps and Imaginations: Sociology Confronts the Genome." *Social Problems* 42, no. 1 (1995): 1–10.

———. "The Products of Conception: The Social Context of Reproductive Choices." *Journal of Medical Ethics* 11 (1985): 188–93.

———. *Recreating Motherhood: Ideology and Technology in a Patriarchal Society.* New York: W. W. Norton, 1989.

———. *The Tentative Pregnancy: Prenatal Diagnosis and the Future of Motherhood.* New York: Viking, 1986.

Rowland, Robyn. "Motherhood, Patriarchal Power, Alienation and the Issue of 'Choice' in Sex Preselection." In *Man-Made Women: How New Reproductive Technologies Affect Women,* ed. Gena Corea et al., 74–87. London: Hutchinson, 1985.

———. "Of Women Born, But for How Long? The Relationship of Women to the New Reproductive Technologies and the Issue of Choice." In *Made to Order: The Myth of Reproductive and Genetic Progress,* ed. Patricia Spallone and Deborah Lynn Steinberg, 67–83. New York: Pergamon Press, 1987.

Ruddick, Sara. "Maternal Thinking." In *Mothering: Essays in Feminist Theory,* ed. Joyce Trebilcot, 213–30. Totowa, N.J.: Rowman & Allanheld, 1983.

Ruether, Rosemary Radford. *Sexism and God-Talk: Toward a Feminist Theology.* Boston: Beacon Press, 1983.

Ryan, Maura A. "The Argument for Unlimited Procreative Liberty: A Feminist Critique." *Hastings Center Report* 20, no. 4 (1990): 6–12.

———. "Feminist Theology and the New Genetics." In *The Ethics of Genetic Engineering,* ed. Maureen Junker-Kenny and Lisa Sowle Cahill, 93–101. London: SCM Press, 1998.

———. "Justice and Artificial Reproduction: A Catholic Feminist Analysis." Ph.D. diss., Yale University, 1993.

———. "The New Reproductive Technologies: Defying God's Dominion?" *Journal of Medicine and Philosophy* 20 (1995): 419–38.

Sarin, A. R. "Women: Half the World — Half the Power." *Journal of Obstetrics, Gynaecology and Family Welfare* 3, no. 14 (1997): 5–11.

Schockenhoff, Eberhard. "First Sheep, Then Human Beings? Theological and Ethical Reflections on the Use of Gene Technology." In *The Ethics of Genetic Engineering,* ed. Maureen Junker-Kenny and Lisa Sowle Cahill, 85–92. London: SCM Press, 1998.

Schulte, Brigid. "Want a Boy? An Age Gap Could Help." *San Jose Mercury News,* September 25, 1997, 6A.

Sen, Amartya. "More Than 100 Million Women Are Missing." *New York Review of Books,* December 20, 1990, 61–66.

Shannon, Thomas A. "Ethical Issues in Genetics." *Theological Studies* 60 (1999): 111–23.

———. *What Are They Saying About Genetic Engineering?* New York: Paulist Press, 1985.

Shinn, Roger Lincoln. *The New Genetics: Challenges for Science, Faith, and Politics.* Wakefield, R.I.: Moyer Bell, 1996.

Sherwin, Susan. "Feminist Ethics and In Vitro Fertilization." In *Science, Morality, and Feminist Theory,* ed. Marsha Hanene and Kai Nielsen, 265–84. Calgary: University of Calgary Press, 1987.

Sinsheimer, Robert L. "The Prospect of Designed Genetic Change." In *Ethics, Reproduction and Genetic Control,* ed. Ruth F. Chadwick, 136–46. New York: Routledge, 1992.

Smith, J. David, and K. Ray Nelson. *The Sterilization of Carrie Buck.* Far Hills, N.J.: New Horizon Press, 1989.

Smith, Janet Farrell. "Parenting and Property." In *Mothering: Essays in Feminist Theory,* ed. Joyce Trebilcot, 199–212. Totowa, N.J.: Rowman & Allanheld, 1983.

Southwick, Karen. "Use Norplant, Don't Go to Jail." *San Francisco Chronicle,* August 2, 1992, Z1/13.

Stanworth, Michelle, ed. *Reproductive Technologies: Gender, Motherhood and Medicine.* Minneapolis: University of Minnesota Press, 1987.

Steinbacher, Roberta. "Should Parents Be Prohibited from Choosing the Sex of Their Child? Yes." *Health* 8, no. 2 (1994): 24.

Steinbacher, Roberta, and Helen B. Holmes. "Sex Choice: Survival and Sisterhood." In *Man-Made Women: How New Reproductive Technologies Affect Women,* ed. Gena Corea et al., 52–63. London: Hutchinson, 1985.

Steinbock, Bonnie, and Ron McClamrock. "When Is Birth Unfair to the Child?" *Hastings Center Report* 24, no. 6 (1994): 15–21.

Stolberg, Sheryl Gay. "Youth's Death Shaking Up Field of Gene Experiments on Humans." *New York Times,* January 27, 2000, A1, A20.

Sutton, Agneta. "The New Genetics: Facts, Fictions and Fears." *Linacre Quarterly* 62, no. 3 (1995): 76–87.

Suzuki, David, and Peter Knudtson. *Genethics: The Ethics of Engineering Life.* Rev. ed. Cambridge, Mass.: Harvard University Press, 1990.

"Tennessee Eyes Reward for Birth Control." *San Francisco Chronicle,* April 17, 1992, A9.

Thompson, Larry. "The First Kids With New Genes." *Time,* June 7, 1993, 50–53.

Timberg, Craig. "Virginia House Regrets 'Eugenics.'" *San Francisco Chronicle,* February 4, 2001, A3, A8.

Tong, Rosemarie. *Feminist Approaches to Bioethics: Theoretical Reflections and Practical Applications.* Boulder, Colo.: Westview Press, 1997.

Traina, Christina L. H. *Feminist Ethics and Natural Law: The End of Anathemas.* Washington, D.C.: Georgetown University Press, 1999.

United Church of Christ. "Pronouncement: Church and Genetic Engineering." In *Minutes of the Seventeenth General Synod,* 42–43. United Church of Christ, 1989.

United States Supreme Court. "Buck v. Bell." In *Contemporary Issues in Bioethics,* ed. Tom L. Beauchamp and LeRoy Walters, 607–8. Belmont, Calif.: Wadsworth, 1994.

Verhey, Allen. "'Playing God' and Invoking a Perspective." *Journal of Medicine and Philosophy* 20 (1995): 347–64.

Vines, Gail. "The Hidden Cost of Sex Selection." *New Scientist* 138, no. 1871 (1993): 12–13.

Wade, Nicholas. "Gene Linked to High I.Q. Is Reported Found with New Technique." *New York Times,* May 14, 1998, A12.

———. "Reports on Human Genome Challenge Long-Held Beliefs." *New York Times,* February 12, 2001, A1, A16.

———. "Scientists Decode Down Syndrome Chromosome." *New York Times,* May 9, 2000, D4.

Walter, James J. "'Playing God' or Properly Exercising Human Responsibility?: Some Theological Reflections on Human Germ-Line Therapy." *New Theology Review* 10, no. 4 (1997): 39–59.

Walters, LeRoy, and Julie Gage Palmer. *The Ethics of Human Gene Therapy*. New York: Oxford University Press, 1997.

Warren, Mary Ann. *Gendercide: The Implications of Sex Selection*. Totowa, N.J.: Rowman & Allanheld, 1985.

Weiss, Rick. "Gene Enhancements' Thorny Ethical Traits." *Washington Post,* October 12, 1997, A1, A18–19.

Wertz, Dorothy C. "Reproductive Technologies: Sex Selection." In *Encyclopedia of Bioethics,* ed. Warren Thomas Reich, rev. ed., 2212–16. New York: Simon & Schuster Macmillan, 1995.

Wertz, Dorothy C., and John C. Fletcher. "Fatal Knowledge? Prenatal Diagnosis and Sex Selection." *Hastings Center Report* 19 (May–June 1989): 21–27.

———. "Sex Selection through Prenatal Diagnosis: A Feminist Critique." In *Feminist Perspectives in Medical Ethics,* ed. Helen Bequaert Holmes and Laura M. Purdy, 240–53. Bloomington and Indianapolis: Indiana University Press, 1992.

Wilmut, Ian. "Dolly's False Legacy." *Time,* January 11, 1999, 74–77.

World Council of Churches. *Manipulating Life: Ethical Issues in Genetic Engineering.* Geneva: World Council of Churches, 1982.

Zambrana, Ruth E. "A Research Agenda on Issues Affecting Poor and Minority Women: A Model for Understanding Their Health Needs." In *Too Little, Too Late: Dealing with the Health Needs of Women in Poverty,* ed. Cesar A. Perales and Lauren S. Young, 137–60. New York: Harrington, 1988.

Zoloth-Dorfman, Laurie. "Mapping the Normal Human Self: The Jew and the Mark of Otherness." In *Genetics: Issues of Social Justice,* ed. Ted Peters, 180–202. Cleveland: Pilgrim Press, 1998.

Index